The Construction And Operation Of Clandestine Drug Laboratories

The Construction And Operation Of Clandestine Drug Laboratories

Second Edition

by Jack B. Nimble

Loompanics Unlimited
Port Townsend, Washington

The Construction And Operation Of Clandestine Drug Laboratories, Second Edition

Published by:
Loompanics Unlimited
PO Box 1197
Port Townsend, WA 98368
Loompanics Unlimited is a division of Loompanics Enterprises, Inc.

Cover by Daniel Wend/MEDIA Graphics
Illustrations by Jack B. Nimble

ISBN 1-55950-108-1
Library of Congress Card Catalog 93-80258

Contents

There is no calamity greater
than lavish desires,
And there is no greater desire
than greed...

The more laws and order are
made prominent, the more
thieves and robbers there
will be...

He who knows others is wise
He who knows himself is enlightened...

People are difficult to govern
because they have too much
knowledge...

—Lao Tzu (from *The Way Of Life*)

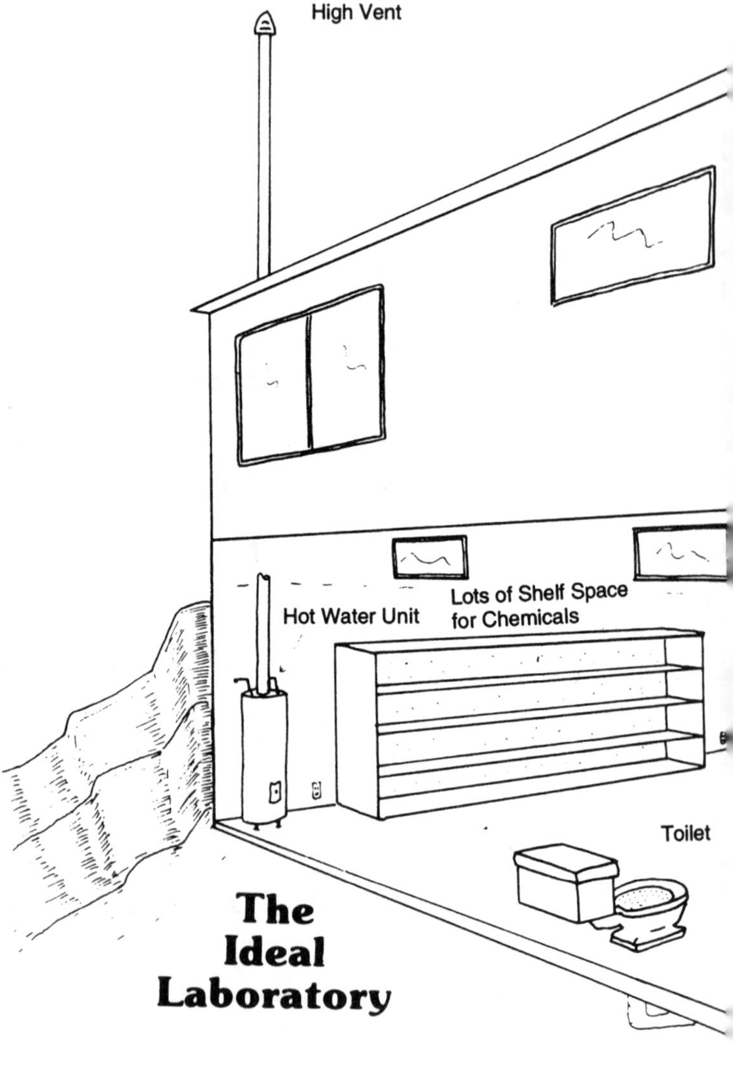

The Ideal Laboratory

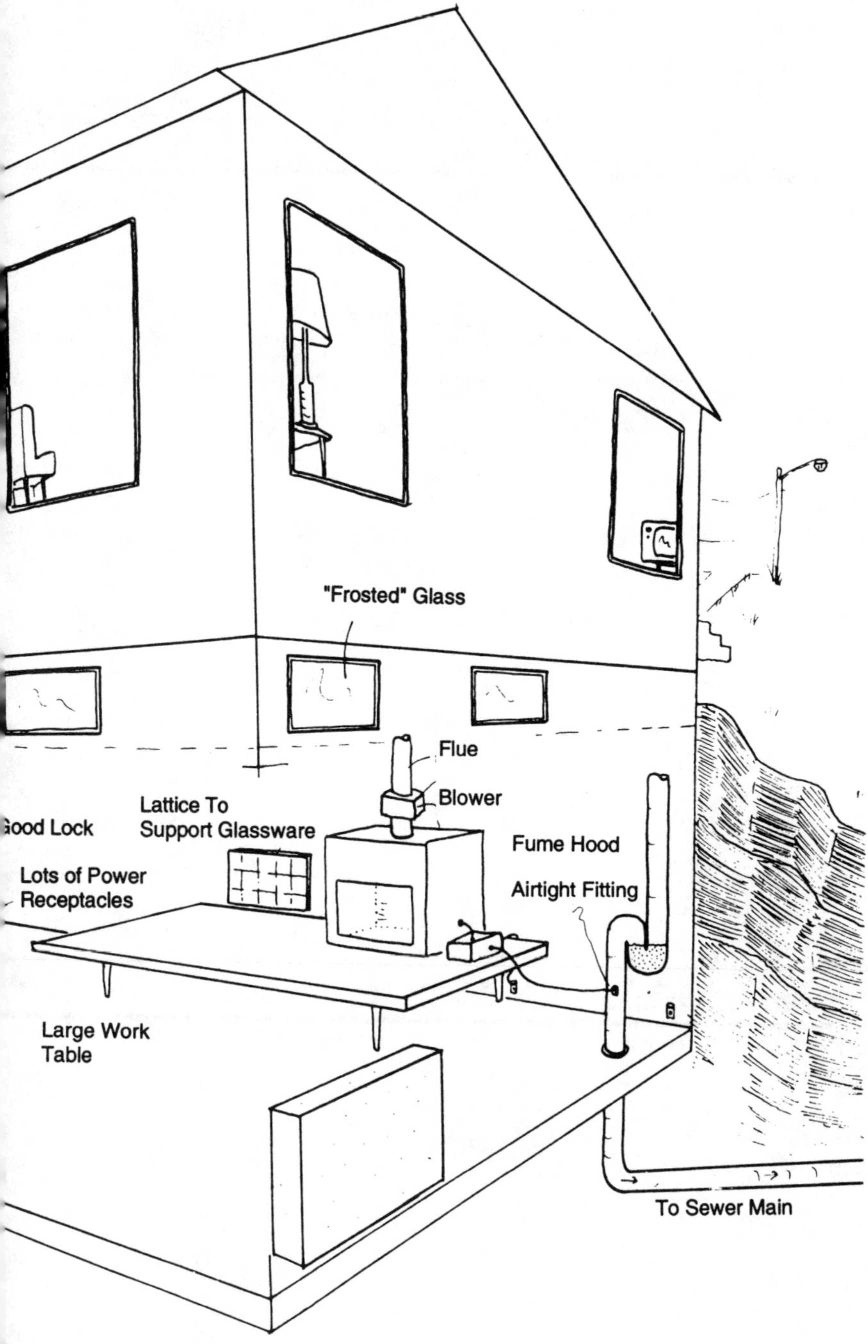
"Frosted" Glass
Flue
Blower
Lattice To
Support Glassware
Good Lock
Fume Hood
Lots of Power
Receptacles
Airtight Fitting
Large Work
Table
To Sewer Main

Preface to the Second Edition

Well, the 1990s are now with us and much has changed since the first edition. The War on Drugs, increasing cooperation of chemical suppliers, product liability-awareness, and stringent new regulations have made operating a clandestine laboratory more challenging (and profitable) than ever.

Sadly, we now live in a world where lawsuits and lobbying legislate regulations and dictate behavior in the business world. This book is sold for *informational purposes only*. The information contained herein is my opinion. I do not encourage anyone to break any law, or violate any local, state, federal, or international statutes, guidelines, regulations, building codes, zoning ordinances, or anything bearing a remote similarity. If you are unsure of the legality of anything you do, or think of doing, or are about to think about doing, I urge you to seek out the authorities and question them!

Please understand this book concerns building and operating a laboratory — it is NOT a book on drug chemistry. Don't ask me how to synthesize things. There are already many good books available in that arena. Michael Valentine Smith's *Psychedelic Chemistry* is one of particular merit. It could use a better index, but it's still excellent. All procedures include scientific literature references, so you can dig up the original publication. For the phenethylamine (amphetamine) class of drugs, Dr. Alexander Shulgin's *Pihkal* is "the book." His philosophy on drugs is illuminating too. I am also grateful to the many persons who have shown me their laboratories in recent years — their ingenuity and mistakes are fully reflected in this edition. If I can be allowed to generalize, these labs seem to divide into two distinct categories. One, you just want to hurry up and get the hell out of before something blows up, or the police dynamite the door. The other kind, you just have a deep down feeling that everything is cool. There are no nasty smells, the property fits in with its surroundings, there isn't powder dried all over the counter top, scores of tin cans everywhere with remnants of "bad batches," or empty chemical containers in the trash with the labels still on them. Which category do you fall into?

I've been criticized on occasion for not presenting the reader with enough specifics. I would like to respond to this. My attempt in this book is to introduce the reader to various ways a clandestine laboratory is built and operated, with a variety of materials and situations. I have included specific examples of how these methods have worked well for myself and others. If you are a person who must have a specific diagram in front of you, listing every part and its exact specifications, as well as instructions that tell instructions that tell you exactly where to buy glass jars and plastic spatulas — you'll probably be dissatisfied with this book. I would be surprised if you ever actually operate a successful clandestine laboratory. I would also guess that you were probably looking for a book that you can pick up and read that will make you an expert chemist. This hobby requires that you be resourceful. You should have things like a chemical compatibility chart on your wall for reference; and, you should be able to recognize the differences between polycarbonate, polyethylene, Teflon, etc. Such knowledge means you don't dissolve that kitchen cup you're about to pour your solution into. I've included many more sources of information in this edition.

Like anything else, you will only become good at chemistry through experience. A degree in chemistry will certainly give you a flying start, but you must learn most of it through experience. Most drug manufacturing procedures fall under the category of "organic chemistry." This means simply the chemistry related to carbon compounds. Organic chemistry is a very seat-of-the-pants type of science. Most of the learning takes place in the laboratory, not on a chalkboard. I have many times duplicated a published procedure *exactly* as described — down to the identical equipment, identical quantities, and same sources of the reagent chemicals — nearly always to find a significant difference in yields, temperatures, reaction times, etc. It is only through experience that you learn to steer a straight path through these perplexing moments with a solid feeling for what is correct procedure.

And let me take a brief moment to interject something that you will probably be surprised to find in an underground-drug publication: a discussion of ethical behavior. You will of course do what you want to do, but let me enlighten you just a tiny bit about "responsibilities."

All drugs are *not* created equal. You must always remember that your fellow humans are trusting you greatly (sometimes ignorantly) when they ingest your creations. It's easy to look at that semi-pure powder and convince yourself it's good enough, and forgo the final rinse or recrystallization. Don't be the brown-powder fool who proclaims: "Hell, man, it never made me sick..." Many people are hypersensitive to the byproducts you neglect to remove from your batch. Of course, you have no control over the *quantity* people will take, if they will abuse it excessively, have a bad trip, freak out, etc. If you manufactured motorcycles, people would buy them and drive like marauders, and, eventually, someone would get hurt on a machine you made. Perhaps it was their recklessness, or perhaps it was that axle nut your assembler forgot to tighten. Perhaps you manufacture kitchen knives? Eventually, *someone* will cut themselves, even use one of them to commit suicide or murder. My point is: you simply have to do the very best that you can do, and always remember that others (many you will never meet) are trusting you greatly. You owe it to all concerned to always deliver consistent purity and dosages.

One final word on this subject: your *choice* of product. Exactly what are you making? Personally, I would have a big problem manufacturing crack, ice, methylfentanyl, etc., for mass distribution and consumption. These are a special breed of drugs that seem to perpetually torment the user and imprison the dealer. Leave these substances to the fools dumb enough to make them. It is my sincere hope that the information I present here is used with good intent. Clandestine chemistry can be grossly profitable. It is unfortunate that good ideals are often lost in the midst of huge profits. This book is for those wonderful people who value freedom and the human spirit above money and power. Perhaps if these people begin to voice their opinions more, the day of responsible drug use, manufacture, and control will become a reality. Enough said.

Manufacturing drugs can involve a certain degree of risk, which varies from country to country. Unfortunately, I have had several acquaintances who have lived through the nightmare of a bust. In this second edition, I share some of their "why and how" stories with you.

This edition also seems to breathe a more militant tone than the first. This is not really intentional. It is simply a reflection of the environment surrounding clandestine labs at this time. The War On Drugs, Inc. has become an entire industry, sucking up billions of dollars and feeding itself with lots of high profile media coverage. Drugs are blamed for everything: poverty, crime, AIDS, even threats to national security. Everyone has seen the crack-house busts on TV, with police agents decked out in full tactical gear and armed with automatic weapons. You've seen them storming into private homes, often with small children inside. They seem to never show one of the 45 percent that end up in no arrests. And you hear them proclaiming loudly that they're winning this "war!" The entire criminal legal system is clogged daily with thousands of minor drug-possession charges. Judges are often handing out 20 years to life for drugs while rape and violent cases settle for less than 5. Even a death penalty for drug "kingpins" has been proposed.

Well, I doubt seriously if things will change anytime soon. I have stopped spending so much time worrying about when the Drug War will be declared a truce, and I have omitted much of my bitter treatise on drug politics from the first edition.

I am not suggesting I have the answer to drug abuse. I wish only to illustrate how the present system consumes valuable resources and worsens the problem, in spite of a few good intentions.

The clandestine laboratories described in this book don't have to be used to make illegal drugs. They could be used to manufacture medicines and useful chemicals in war or survival situations. This book contains what I know about setting up and operating clandestine laboratories. *It is sold for informational purposes only.*

The Risks

Throughout this book I put great emphasis on the DEA, and less on local enforcement agencies. Why? If you're a careful, proficient chemist, you probably won't get busted... the odds are tipped in your favor. But if you do, even though you're careful and proficient, it will probably be from a lead developed through your chemical (or lab equipment) suppliers, which generally cooperate with the DEA rather than local units. If you are a sloppy crank lab, your neighbors will think you look suspicious and call the local police. They'll come out, go through your trash looking for clues, probably find some, probably smell your lab, and even go in on probable cause. If you are busted as a result of a larger investigation working its way backwards from some street dealer who plea-bargained, it could be the DEA, or perhaps a local task force. Most communities have these task forces, (which are part of the local police network), set up for the specific purpose of performing drug-related raids. Many of them are trained and equipped like the Green Berets or Special Forces. They enter premises with battering rams that will break solid concrete, shoot tear-gas and noise makers in through the windows, and use automatic weapons. If you find yourself trying to "prepare" yourself for an encounter with these guys, then I seriously question your sanity and intelligence. Not being discovered in the first place is the only sensible place to put your efforts.

Never underestimate forensic science when you think you're disposing of evidence. Fingerprints, traces of saliva, hair, skin cells, foot prints, nearly anything you deal with can be traced back to you. There is no way to eliminate all the holes. The most important thing is not getting discovered in the first place. Keep traces of drugs off the things you throw in the trash, or anything else that will be accessible to other people (even envelopes and paper!). There are cases on the books where agents scraped the residue of a drug intermediate (even precursors) out of containers that chemists have left outside or thrown away. This evidence easily leads to probable cause.

Most drug users, dealers, and manufacturers are sent to state penitentiaries. In a few cases, such as federal tax evasion, money laundering, federal analog laws, and similar federal raps you *may* go to a federal prison. These are a bit better, as a general rule. But don't count on it just because you're manufacturing some exotic analog. You'll probably still spend time in a hell-hole state facility.

Fortunately, as of this writing, the justice system is being forced to release non-violent/non-repeat offenders to make room in crowded prisons. This is just one more reason not to have lots of guns and ammo laying around in your lab.

Prison is a horrible environment to spend your life in. It's even a horrible place to visit someone you know. Fortunately, I have never spent a single night in a jail cell, but I've talked with and visited many who have, a couple of them very good friends. I will share a few of their stories with you. I have changed only the names and places, to protect their actual identities.

Blake had been a clandestine chemist off and on for several years. Though careless sometimes, he generally knew what he was doing and took the time to understand chemical reactions and achieve precision in his work. He had a solid background in sciences, and was an excellent user of libraries and other research aids. He had made good profits in previous years from several mega-large batches. Bored one summer, he decided on another "final" batch, utilizing some of the chemicals he had left, but ordering more primary precursors. His old supply leads proved to be okay again, and he received his orders without incident. Cash in hand, he rented a large farm in a tiny rural community. He spent very little time on the farm, visiting only once or twice a month, usually entertaining friends with "product." The final big batch turned into many little ones. While away, a nosy landlord entered the property, and noticed empty chemical containers along the side of a barn. He wrote down the names of all the chemicals and took them to the sheriff. The sheriff turned that information over to the local police and with a few phone calls they quickly surmised exactly what he was making. The investigation was snowballing already. Several spills around the property were also analyzed and proved to have either traces of drugs or intermediates. Probable cause galore! They waited for days, watching the place like hawks — video cameras, night-vision scopes, etc. They let him return, watched him a few days until they determined he was manufacturing, and raided. He had everything right there — precursors, labware with his fingerprints all over it, gallons of wastes (indicating previous activity), notes, product, etc. It was all over. He spent most of his legal slush fund trying to convince the local court that he was at least one step above a child pornographer. In a larger city, he faced a court of appeals, almost penniless, with disastrous results. He is currently serving a 15 year sentence.

Michael was a true researcher. He made drugs of all types simply for the chance to try something exotic. He kept detailed notes on many of the never-before-taken substances he made. He didn't really need the money, but it brought in a lot anyway.

Michael had an attorney on retainer since his entry into the illicit drug business. And this proved worthwhile, at least partly. Like Blake, he moved his operation to a remote farm, one owned by his family. He pulled off several gargantuan batches of various exotic drugs there, then kicked back and enjoyed life awhile. A year later, he opted for a final "one last batch." Indeed it was his last batch. An old acquaintance from down south showed up one day. They talked about the good old days when he used to burn up his kitchen. His acquaintance told him of a friend that worked for a chemical company that had an "inside line" on anything he needed. Michael was delighted! An introduction was arranged.

The guy arrived a week later with his acquaintance. They all ate dinner together, and Michael began to feel he could trust this guy. He spoke the same language, reminiscing about old drug tales. What Michael did not know was that this guy with an inside line was a DEA agent, and his old acquaintance had offered information on him as part of a plea bargain to get out of a methamphetamine possession charge in another state. He was raided at 5:00 AM in the morning, just as the birds were beginning to sing.

At first it looked as if his attorney had been successful — he was immediately out on bail, and the prosecution failed to prove probable cause. But the DEA wasn't giving up, and they had the taxpayers' resources to fight the case down to stems and seeds! He fled, a penniless fugitive, before his final court date. He has never been seen since.

Dana was with Robert as he made a batch, like so many times before. They left for a few days to take a break. The two of them were busted together in their house/lab after the landlord noticed water running out the garage door, and went in "in good faith" to repair the leak. They returned to find an unwelcome party waiting. Robert fled before his court date, leaving Dana to face charges alone. Her attorney attempted to prove that she was not aware of his activities, but her fingerprints were all over the glassware and counter surfaces. She was released after serving four years of a 15 year sentence. This bust could have been avoided altogether if the lab had been more obscure.

Coby was a dealer for many years before he dipped his wick into the clandestine manufacturing business. Four years later he was busted with evidence leading back nearly three years, and involving over 300 hours of telephone tapping, including many cellular telephone taps. The obvious message from his situation is that way too many people were involved.

A trip to a law library will yield many hours of interesting reading about drug cases. Many of the cases will surprise you, often the simplest, most absurd mistakes led to the bust.

Security

One of the finest skills to master is silence. Unconditional silence. Mistakes made here will cost you time in the slammer, maybe even your life. I cannot stress enough how important anonymity is.

I have backed off a bit from my stance in the first edition that anything but a one-person operation is insane. That's unrealistic. At some point or another you will have to deal with someone else in the course of business. Just use these reminders as guidelines: Few chemical procedures require more than two hands. Working alone means no one to snitch on you later. It also means no one to argue profits and operations with, and no one to scam some of the harvest while you're not watching. Few chemists, if any, are caught who truly act alone. The many voices of experience echo: "work alone." But working with someone is fun, and it makes for great conversation and stories a few years later when you're sitting around having a beer:

> "*...that time when we dumped that 55 gallon batch down the drain thinking it was waste... and that time we improvised the outboard motor for an emergency stirrer... and that time the landlord walked in the back door, and that time we...*"

Security also means unobtrusive behavior on your part. Cover all your tracks. Have good ruses ready for any nosy person. If a neighbor complains about an odor, say you spilt some carburetor cleaner or plating bath or something else like that. Act as if the smells are equally noxious to yourself, say "sorry," and shut down completely for a while. Never leave glassware, empty chemical containers, chemistry books, or lab equipment in sight of others. Do not ever *ever* have chemicals or lab equipment sent to your residence or place of manufacture. Postal and DOT regulations require conspicuous warning labels on many chemical shipments. Packages are often left with neighbors if you're not home. Also, never leave these empty shipping containers out on the curb or alley to be taken off as trash. Tear off all labels, put them in opaque trash bags and throw them in a dumpster across town.

Always completely eliminate visibility into your working area. Police now routinely use video cameras and night-vision scopes to obtain search warrant evidence. Frosted glass is good, and allows light to enter. The spray-on glass frosting has a tendency to flake off. A white curtain lets light in, and blocks the view even if the window is broken. Aluminum foil is overkill and looks suspicious. I've seen some people put up a curtain then fasten a flat black piece of plywood behind that. From the outside, it looks like a normal room with the lights off all the time. It also provides protection against anyone entering through the window.

Perform smelly distillations and evaporations during late hours when most people are asleep, and do them under a fume hood. Foul weather is another good time as few persons will be outside. Rain also has the remarkable ability to cleanse the air of odors. The chapter on fume hoods discusses the elimination of odors in detail. Beware when working with ether. Its strong and distinctive odor has blown the cover of many clandestine labs. It's also *extremely* flammable. Use an alternate solvent unless you have the proper equipment and facilities. Ether is a smelly, dangerous solvent. I discuss ether in more detail in a later chapter.

Keep drugs out of your laboratory. Store them in a secure, obscure, and confidential place after manufacture. *Thoroughly* wash all glassware and equipment with a good detergent. Follow with an acetone (or similar) rinse afterwards. Your tax dollars have purchased elaborate, expensive equipment that forensic narcs use to detect molecular-sized traces of most drugs. Don't ever underestimate the prowess of forensic chemists! The World Trade Center bombing in 1993 was a good example of how much information is buried in residual evidence, even after an explosion. People who tell you that setting your lab on fire (to destroy evidence) when you hear the doors being kicked in are not informed. You'll only add an arson charge to your legal troubles.

Watch spills — clean them up thoroughly. Don't leave drugs in various stages of production laying around to be completed "later." Finish up, clean-up, and get the stuff out of your laboratory. Be able to pack up your entire operation (chemicals and fancy equipment, that is) on a moment's notice. Have with you at any given time only the chemicals and equipment you need for a given procedure.

Know where the toilet is, and be prepared to dispose of as much contraband as possible on a second's warning. Even though you may still have evidence around, you'll be much better off in court with 0.23 grams than with 2 pounds.

Watch for surveillance too. Physical surveillance is not hard to spot if you continuously look for it. Cars, vans, and recreational vehicles are notorious as tools of surveillance used by narcs. Wire taps and pen registers are common as well. *Never* discuss *any* aspect of drugs on *your* telephone. Avoid suspicious innuendoes and lingo too. Should you suspect surveillance, stop *then*. Cease operation for several months. Surveillance is very expensive. It involves a lot of time from highly paid persons. Even pen registers (a listing of all numbers dialed on a particular phone) require much time and money to analyze. For these reasons, surveillance is usually ceased if positive evidence is not being produced. Be irregular. Never make promises about exact delivery times, sales, etc. Maintain the ability to stop at any time. The added margin of security is well worth any inconveniences from an irregular schedule. Think ahead and you won't be sorry later — and *always* consider very carefully taking on a partner.

What are the communication requirements of the clandestine chemist, and how can they be safely satisfied? Later I will discuss the use of an answering service. Never give a chemical company your home telephone number, or any other number that can be traced directly to you. Finding to whom a particular telephone number belongs is a simple phone call for any local, state, or federal official. You must also be very selective about whom you place calls to from your phone, as this information (the actual numbers that you dial) is also readily available without a warrant. Caller-ID is available in many areas, displaying your number on someone's phone before they even answer it! This is where a handful of quarters and a payphone with some privacy are important. Be sure to prepay more time than you ever expect to use. It would be awful to have a recording say, "You have one minute left, please deposit 75 cents for three additional minutes," just as you were closing that deal on 20 lbs of a hard to get precursor.

Few persons know exactly how many wiretaps are made each year, and while I personally suspect the number is small, you should *always* assume that everything you say on the telephone is being monitored. The consequences of an unknown phone tap are usually devastating. And what about cellular phones? While they may provide a degree of ambiguity regarding the exact origin of a call, they are more easily monitored, and present fewer legal obstacles for the authorities to intercept. In fact, there is an entire hobby developing in this country of monitoring cellular and portable phones. More than once, the police have gotten solid leads and developed usable evidence based on the numbers stored in confiscated cellular phones (and pagers). Nearly all cellular phones remember the last number you dialed so you can use a "redial" button. Also, a new technology known as "cellular mapping" has recently become available that allows the location of a cellular phone to be generalized, even the movement from "cell" to "cell" as a moving caller progresses. The most disturbing thing of all is that they can apply this type of "trace" to calls made months (even years!) ago, using the information the telephone company can provide. The bottom line? Try to use telephones of any type (and pagers) as little as possible. When you must use them, use pay telephones.

Drug laboratories are busted all the time. The typical scenario is a speed lab in a garage with dozens of jars laying around, no exhaust fan, empty drums in the alley, souped-up cars in the driveway, etc. Watch the news and you can learn from others' mistakes.

Often, busts occur because of the lab's audacity, not from a police investigation. I was watching the news recently, and a laboratory in Los Angeles was busted when neighbors noticed noxious yellow smoke seeping out from under the garage door. The fire department was called, and they were inside the garage before the resident even knew they were there. Inside was really a mess: loose exposed wires, clutter all over the floor and dozens of half-full chemical jars. If you have a fire or other disaster, it is usually legal for emergency crews to enter by force, and any evidence found is considered obtained in "good faith." Keep everything neat and clean. Believe me, I tried it all different ways, and neatness *always* works best. You'll make more product, you'll be under less stress while you work, and you'll sleep better at night.

Similar circumstances arise if your place is burglarized or vandalized. This problem is compounded if you have a monitored alarm that goes off. I would stay away from alarms. The best insurance is to keep the lab hidden even from a burglar that's already inside. A heavy door and lock are a must. My favorite deadbolt is the nearly pick-and-drill-proof Medico. Combined with a steel door they provide a very secure passageway. Don't forget windows either. Frosted glass is great, but suppose someone throws a rock through the window? Is your lab still out of view or is a giant peephole now visible from across the street, right into your workspace?

Out in the country, a large dog (or two) are great for keeping people away from your operation. No one is likely to smell anything if they can never get closer than 500 yards to your lab. In the city, they are great to have inside while you are gone, to prevent burglary. Even the most desperate soul will not likely enter the premises should they hear barking inside. My personal favorite lab dog is the Rottweiler. Their appearance is very intimidating, they become very attached to their "pack" (you), and they seem to naturally develop a "protect and serve" disposition. Like no other breed, they can smell out trouble. Females are especially loyal. For a lab dog, seek one that is laid-back and not hyper. Treat your dog well, and never ever let them "sample the batch." Dogs are much more sensitive to many drugs than humans, and probably wouldn't enjoy it anyway. Besides, you want them on their toes to listen for intruders. They're also great company, help calm your nerves, don't rat on you later, and don't really care if what you're doing is legal or not. I recommend dogs.

Safety and security are tightly related. Take a look around and ask yourself, "What is the worst disaster that could happen here?" And then ask, "Could it contain itself?" Ideally, your lab has a high ceiling, concrete or brick walls and a cement floor with a drain. Kept clean, this environment will handle all but the biggest mishaps without taking your house with it. One fairly new product to hit the market in recent years are the self-contained Halon fire extinguishers. These units mount against the ceiling, or inside a cabinet. They are equipped with a fuse that melts at 160 degrees F. They then flood the area with Halon gas, which quickly quenches nearly any type of fire and leaves no residue — so you might even salvage your batch. Afterwards, they're refillable. Make sure you get one for the proper size area you wish to protect (their capacity is rated in cubic feet), and remember they only work best in enclosed places. So keep one or two inside your fume hood, another inside your flammable solvents cabinet, etc. They are cheap insurance. At least consider a large manually operated Halon extinguisher.

Anyone who has experienced a clandestine laboratory fire knows what an absolutely terrifying experience it is. It usually happens very suddenly, and as you struggle frantically to get it under control your mind is racing through many thoughts. Is it bad enough to call the fire department? Should I try to destroy as much evidence as I can first? What can I tell them this place is? Should I just get out now while I can, and before my solvent cabinet explodes? The entire scenario runs its course in minutes, even seconds — your life and freedom are put right on the line. You might die, you might go to jail, you might lose your lab and all possessions, or you might put it out, continue your synthesis and be just fine. I have experienced one fire, and that wised me up quickly. I vowed never to put myself through that trauma again. A real gray-hair grower.

Also on the subject of security, I have included the details of an engineering marvel. This device is a kick-in proof, battering-ram proof door that an enterprising gentleman has constructed. This sort of rubbed me the wrong way at first, as I think efforts should go into not being discovered in the first place. But I was so impressed with this device I just have to share it with you (see Figure 1).

From the outside, this door looks rather innocuous. But the secret lies on the other side. It still requires a firmly seated jamb, so I wouldn't recommend it in a wood frame house. The jamb (frame) of this door is fitted with many automobile valve springs that absorb the impact of any blows and return it instantly to its original position. This one was constructed with a rather thin ($^1/_8$ inch) piece of steel as a cover for an ordinary wood door. Angle iron was used to reinforce it from the back. We tested it, and the door won. Using a 3 inch pipe 5 feet long and filled with cement, we rammed and rammed until we could ram no more! We marred the surface of his door up quite a bit, though no structural damage occurred whatsoever. A door like this could buy you some precious time to dispose of contraband until they figured another way into your place. This door is the only thing like it I've ever seen. People who just reinforce a door with steel often find out that a battering ram will punch the whole door right through a brick wall — there's nothing to absorb the energy. I'm sure many improvements could be made to the

design of this door. This same gentleman was already working on a "cutting-torch proof" door! If he's successful, and I ever see him again, I'll share his ingenuity with you again in a future edition.

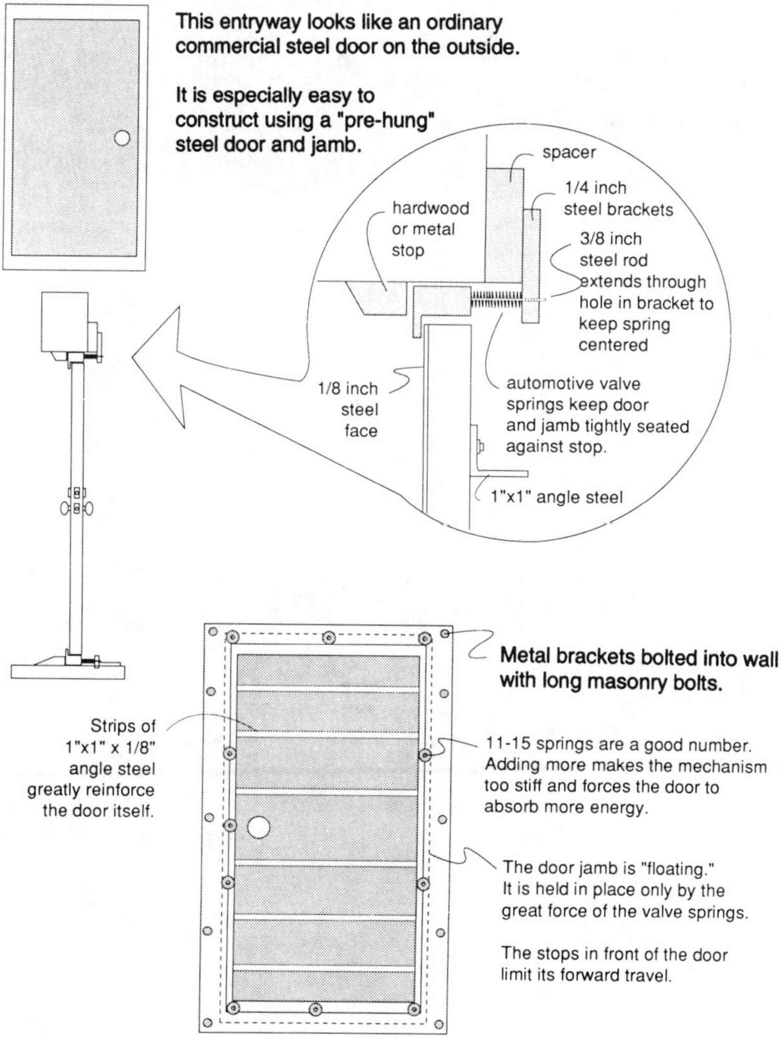

Figure 1

Scanners and Monitoring Equipment

I've been monitoring the DEA's communications for nearly seven years now. (In fact, I am listening to them as I write this!) And how things have changed the past three years! Back in the old days you could eavesdrop on their every move — in fact, an acquaintance I know of avoided a bust entirely because of scanner monitoring. But they are more careful about what they say over the airwaves now. And Motorola now manufactures digital encryption equipment that provides live, real-time scrambling of their most sensitive communications. Even more unfortunate for the clandestine operator are the recent advancements in Low Probability of Interception (LPI) radio. One of these LPI advancements is "spread-spectrum" radio. In this mode the radio's frequency changes randomly several times per second across a wide range of frequencies —

even across an entire band! The receiving radio knows which frequencies to constantly switch to from a random seed number that is sent the instant the microphone is keyed. This technology is the future of government radio. Perhaps in combination with digital encryption it may very well be the ultimate in airwave security. Another LPI technology is "trunking." This mode resembles cellular telephone technology in that the radios hop from frequency to frequency based on their proximity to numerous antennas spaced across the locality. And like cellular phones, they put out very little power (usually less than one watt). So unless you are close to the unit, you will not hear it.

But I told you I was listening to them as I wrote this. How? Well, several big problems remain for government agencies. First is money. This decade is one of declining budgets and tightening of belts. Spread spectrum radio equipment is *very* expensive, and it takes a highly trained (and highly paid) technician to install, program, and maintain it. Even Motorola's digital encryption (DES/DVP) equipment is expensive, and costly to maintain. Trunked radio systems are cheaper, and they are somewhat harder to intercept than standard equipment, but they must maintain close proximity to their antenna network, and they can be monitored most easily if they are in close proximity. This allows the clandestine operator not only to monitor their transmissions when close to your lab (the most important time to listen anyway!) but also to determine *when* they are close to your operation (even if scrambled). If you hear encryption on a trunked frequency, I would start flushing quick!

I definitely hear more encryption, but surprisingly little for how long the technology has been available. Encryption sounds like unmodulated static for the length of the transmission, followed by a short high pitched "beeeep." Interestingly, they often encrypt only one side of the transmission. Often too, they don't seem to know their encryption mode is not on. Coupled with a voice activated tape-recorder (these cost less than 50 dollars) you are provided with a concise synopsis of their daily communications and activities, the portion you are monitoring, that is. I highly recommend scanners.

Most DEA radio activity will be found between 418 and 419 Mhz. They also operate some in the 162.5 to 163.7 range. I have heard them a couple of times in the 417.400 to 418.000 range. IRS and other federal agents like to hang out around 415 to 418 Mhz. Most good scanners allow you to search between an upper and lower frequency limit. The trunking radio systems, which really are not very common, will be found above and below the standard cellular telephone frequencies. Most large cities (even many small ones) have a scanner monitoring club that publishes a listing for that area. Such a list is a good place to start, but remember that the Feds change their frequencies often and it may not be up to date. One nice thing is that scanner monitoring is a perfectly legitimate (and popular!) hobby — there's no need to be shy when asking questions down at the local radio store. Most scanner buffs are conservative, upstanding, voting citizens! Really good scanners have a "search and store" feature that compiles a database of activity and the frequency it occurred on — all while completely unattended!

My recommendations for scanners? Good basic units are Radio Shack's higher end "Pro-" series (the "PRO-2006," "PRO-43," etc.). They scan fast, and cover the new 800 mhz band. They go on sale often for 100 dollars or more off. For a bit more money, the Ace AR-2500, at 500 dollars is an excellent radio. It receives everything from shortwave to 1500 mhz... no gaps. And it has an RS-232 port on the back. This allows you to hook the unit up to a personal computer and do such things as search and store and logging. For instance, when the scanner stops on a specific frequency, your computer screen can instantly log the frequency/date/time/length of the transmission, tell you if you've heard stuff on this frequency before, and if you have, display any notes (example: "DEA ch. 2, local Los Angeles") you have on it.

Also good, though a bit dated, is the ICOM R-7000. It has a built-in search and store mode, not requiring the connection of a computer (although it has an RS-232 port should you want one for some of the bells and whistles mentioned earlier).

A base antenna mounted outside is a must. You wouldn't believe the difference you'll notice from the telescoping antenna that comes with most radios. Base antennas are cheap (less than 20 dollars), and you should mount it as high as you can without it being obtrusive. I have mine painted dark flat brown and stuck up in a tall tree. It's invisible even when you're looking for it.

Whatever you decide to do, don't ever let your scanner give you a false sense of security. NEVER assume that you are hearing all there is to hear; you most certainly are not. Use scanners as just another information gathering tool in your quest to take the fewest risks you can.

Safety

Dangers inherent to organic chemistry cannot be ignored. An accident is an excellent way to draw attention (from friends if you're lucky, from the police if you're not).

Strong acids and bases can severely burn skin. They can also easily blind you. Safety goggles are cheap insurance against the loss of your valuable eyes. Neoprene gloves offer excellent protection from most chemicals. If you have large amounts of concentrated acids, bases, or reactive reagents, transfer working quantities into smaller containers for use in your immediate working area. If a procedure requires a diluted solution, perform the dilution away from other chemicals. Be very careful doing reduction reactions with chemicals like lithium aluminum hydride. When a procedure calls for the maintenance of a low temperature or an inert atmosphere, don't compromise! Hydrogen peroxide, especially above 20 percent concentration, is extremely harmful to your eyes. Concentrated ammonia is also dangerous. It can often be replaced by another, less noxious base, like NaOH or KOH.

Ether seems to always present dangers in a clandestine lab. Learn to respect this highly volatile solvent. Its vapors are heavier than air and can travel downwards to an ignition source. Eliminate all sources of sparks in the area. Florescent lamps, thermostats, telephones, motors, clocks, non-mercury switches, breaker boxes, and relays are notorious sources of ether ignition. The thermostats on many "laboratory" hot-plates spark. Steam baths with a remote source of steam are the safest source of heat if you're using ether. Never store ether in the freezer or refrigerator to retard evaporation! The sparks from the fan or thermostat will cause a violent explosion. Even static charges can trigger ignition. (There *are* very expensive, specially designed freezers for storing flammable solvents, but I won't get into them here.) All conduit, cases, and metal housing should be well grounded. A fume hood is a must for this solvent. Be very careful around ether, if you really must use it at all. It can often be replaced by methylene chloride, chloroform, methyl ethyl ketone, or others as a reaction medium. Its high volatility, sweet aroma and low toxicity make it best suited as a final rinse for many drugs.

Acetone is another popular, flammable solvent that most labs find it hard to be without. Acetone can sometimes be ignited by traveling through the air at high velocity. For this reason, never pour it through the air from a high distance. Even more dangerous is pumping it from one container to another and letting it fall into the bottom of a 55 gallon container. This is especially pertinent to large scale operations. Whenever trucks or railroad cars are filled with acetone, they are pumped with a tube that extends all the way to the bottom of the tank so that no solvent flies through the air. My pals at the solvents supply house educated me about acetone. Very flammable.

A few more suggestions: use pull ties to secure loose cords you might trip over. Never leave a heating operation unattended, especially during evaporation of solvents. And, keep a good fire extinguisher near by and keep it charged.

I doubt seriously if clandestine labs contribute significantly to global pollution, but you can reduce the impact to your own yard and water table. Large manufacturing companies dump all their crap into rivers or leaky underground tanks, or they bribe public officials. Fortunately, as a relatively small operator (compared to say, Bayer) you do not have to use these measures. The media loves to pump up the public's anger when they show drug lab busts on TV. They zoom in the cameras on a spot of dead grass and say, "The owner of *this* lab dumped acid and toxic poisons on the ground... just 500 feet from where *your* children play!"

Always neutralize your waste with lye or muriatic acid (whichever is appropriate) to pH 7. If you have both acidic and basic wastes, consider using them to partially neutralize each other (then use lye or acid to finish). Using a rotary evaporator, or even a simple, home-made "still" can greatly extend the use of your solvents. It simply makes no sense to set a volatile solvent outside to evaporate when you could dry it faster with a still, AND recapture pure, clean solvent for use again. You'll spend less money, breathe fewer fumes, and make fewer risky trips to the chemical store. Reclaimed solvents are as good (often better, more pure) than new ones.

Safety is not only critical for the prevention of injury. It's also important for maintaining secrecy. Think ahead!

Location and Facilities

Most of us lack the financial resources required to construct an ideal laboratory. A large commercial building with a basement on a three-hundred acre secluded lot would be great. But more than likely, your laboratory will be a compromise between what is available and what you can afford.

Basements are wonderfully suited. Water and drain lines are easily accessible. Walls and floors are usually concrete, which is non-flammable and easy to keep clean. Basements are also easily concealed from the rest of the building or house. Persons unfamiliar with the particular building may not even know a basement exists. The entrance door can be made to look like an ordinary closet (with a lock on it, of course). Sounds are deadened.

Windows are usually minimal. And security is usually easier.

With careful planning, however, you can put a lab nearly anywhere. Security and safety are of course the primary concerns when looking for a location. A large, walk-in closet could even work if only small quantities were being dealt with. A garage is good too, provided you have private access. Whatever the location, be certain of several things before you begin or sign a lease. First, that the area is accessible only to you. Don't locate the lab in a place others will walk through to get to circuit breakers or other areas. Be sure visibility is impossible from any window, angle, hole, door, etc. Make certain that adequate arrangements are made for the safe and thorough removal of fumes and odors. Be certain that running water is available (a 5-gallon jug of distilled water can be elevated above the work area and tapped with a siphon). Also, have a toilet (or large drain with water supply) nearby to dispose of products in an "emergency." Last, be absolutely certain you can lock up the lab securely while you're not there, *and* while you're inside working. Ample room is nice if you can have it. I once constructed a small laboratory in the pantry of a tiny bathroom. It was well organized and even had a fume hood built into one of the shelves. I tripped over one of the power cords, jerking a hot plate and beaker of nearly completed product to the floor. This lab never produced a gram of usable product. Don't crowd yourself.

I particularly discourage anyone from putting a lab in an apartment building. Thin walls, neighbors on all sides — it just doesn't make sense. Locate a house, a farm, a small commercial building, a workshop or some thing similar if you plan to do any serious work. Commercial property has an added plus in that you can blend in easier. In any city's industrial district there are always people loading and unloading drums, creating foul odors, and working late hours. I must admit, it's hard for me to enter any establishment without envisioning its use as a clandestine lab. I often enter places that could easily be making drugs right in front of me and I'd never know: people carrying bottles and drums, horrid smells, etc. These places operate every day of the week, year after year, and no one questions a thing. There is no reason you can't operate a clandestine lab with a similar facade.

Wherever you choose, always rent or lease. It will be confiscated from you if you're busted and you own it. And never pay your landlord in cash, it will arouse suspicion. Get a bank money order from the same bank each time and pay at the same time each month. You'll be in like Flynn this way!

35

When to Stop and How

Someone once asked me if I had ever come "close" to getting caught. This doesn't normally happen unless you're very lucky. If you are suspected of illicit manufacture or distribution, you are investigated and apprehended as soon as possible. Since the first edition, there seems to be less and less required to obtain a judge's grant of a search warrant. Such "evidence" can even be a lie from an informant they've cut a deal with. If you make a consistent effort to eliminate evidence of all types, you'll have no regrets.

Several years ago I made the mistake of working with a partner who had "less than sealed" lips. That realization came when I was approached by a third person who claimed they heard I was a "chemist," and asked if I knew of a "recipe" for crank. That was the time to stop, and I did. I was later able to bring that bad "rumor" to an end.

If anyone but you becomes involved or informed, it is time to stop. If you are working with a partner, then things are a bit more complicated. Regardless, if you ever hear something about yourself from someone you didn't tell it to, a big red flag should stand up! If you're asked any unusual questions by anyone that imply "chemical manufacture," consider stopping. If neighbors complain of bad smells, stop. If your precursor shipment was accidently signed for by someone who knows your real identity (i.e., a neighbor), stop. If your answering service gets odd calls, stop. If just about anything happens, stop! Get rid of any products (which you shouldn't have around much anyway), wash up glassware and equipment, and lay low a few months.

History tells that too few clandestine chemists *do* stop. Many get right out of jail and immediately start manufacturing again. I know of numerous individuals either on the run or incarcerated because they didn't stop — most of them in spite of blatant warning signals. Either proceed with your operation flawlessly or pack up. If someone is on to you, it's just a matter of time. This is the voice of experience.

It's a also a great idea to stop frequently anyway — even when things seem to be going well. An ongoing, continuous operation is usually a time bomb.

Glassware

Though you can (and should) use almost any glass containers, you will probably need to purchase a few scientific glassware products. This is the major expense of a laboratory, as most persons lack the expertise to construct such equipment. A good glassware kit is essential. It enables you to efficiently distill substances under reduced pressure, and monitor precise temperatures. These capabilities are essential. Vacuum distillation is a far cry from boiling off unwanted components in a saucepan using a meat thermometer. The typical glassware set also contains equipment to accurately add controlled amounts of one component to another, under inert conditions if necessary. Under vacuum, solvents and reagents can be quickly evaporated and the fumes discharged in a safe manner. Good glassware also facilitates the separation of needed chemicals from commercially available products (this is discussed in more detail later). High quality distillation equipment is the centerpiece of a drug laboratory. This is even more important now than when the first edition was published, because of the unavailability of many chemicals. Good distillation equipment permits the recycling of solvents, sparing you the high-risk affair of purchasing large quantities of solvent.

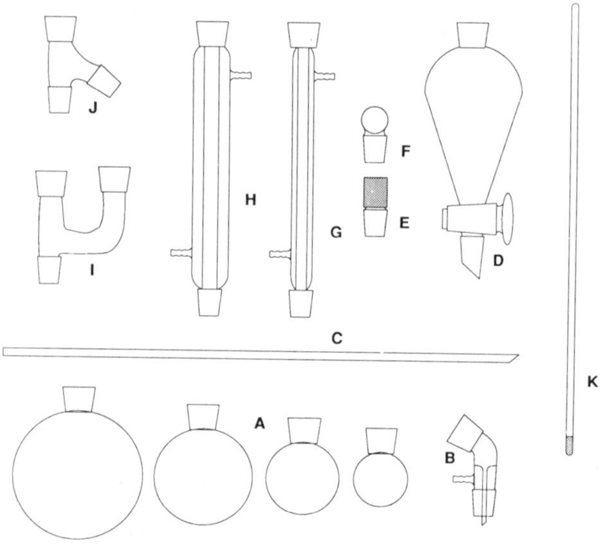

A. Flasks: 25-500 ml
B. Vacuum Adapter
C. Gas Inlet Tube
D. Separatory Funnel
E. Thermometer Adapter
F. Ground Glass Stopper
G. Distillation Column
H. West Condenser
I. Claisen Adapter
J. Connecting Adapter
K. Thermometer

Figure 2

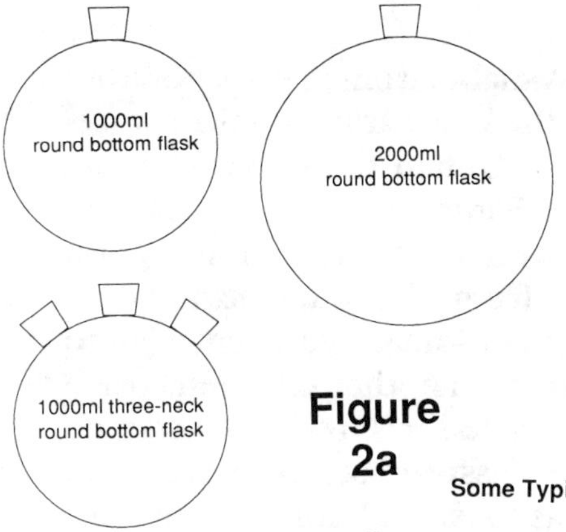

Figure 2a

Some Typical Setups for Drug Syntheses

(Consult an Organic Chemistry lab manual for many more possibilities)

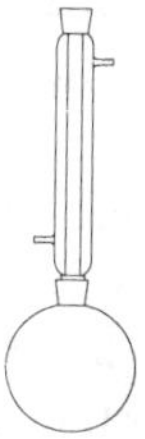

Reflux. This setup is used for reactions which must be gently boiled for long periods of time. Evaporated liquid is returned to the boiling flask.

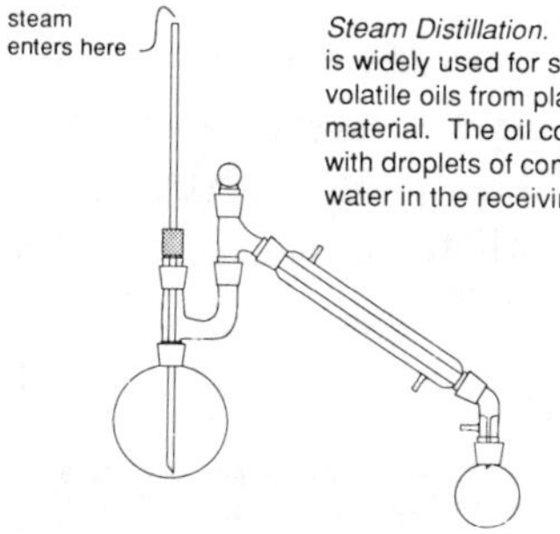

Steam Distillation. This is widely used for separating volatile oils from plant material. The oil comes over with droplets of condensed water in the receiving flask.

Figure 2b

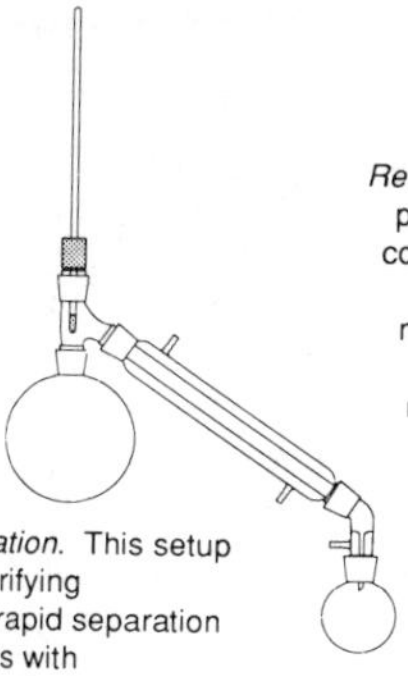

Simple Distillation. This setup is used for purifying solvents and rapid separation of components with widely differing boiling points.

Reflux With Addition. This popular setup allows the controlled addition of one liquid to another, while monitoring temperature. An inert gas such as nitrogen is often bled in from the 3rd neck, if needed. A magnetic stirrer is often used as well.

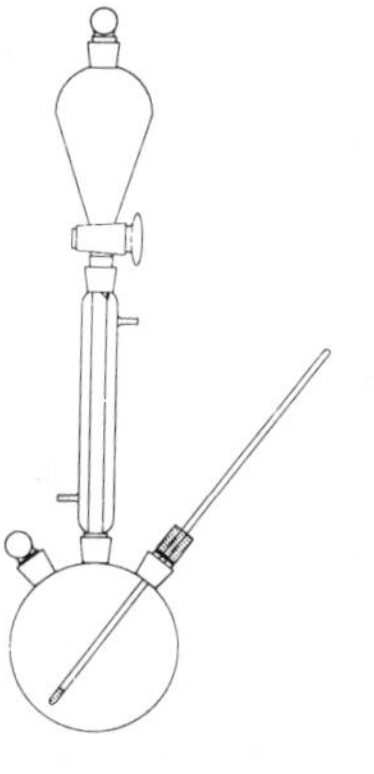

These glassware kits are available from many laboratory supply outlets. I've also seen them at paraphernalia smokeshops at outrageous mark-ups. Obtain the universal type, with ground glass joints (see Figure 2). If you can't find one, browse a current journal (at the library) on "laboratories." You'll find ads from glassware manufacturers as well as sources of other equipment you may wish to invest in. The *Thomas Register* is another excellent place to look, and nearly every library has it. Obtain an accurate thermometer for use with the glassware set. Be certain you know the submersion it was designed for. Seventy-five millimeters (75mm) is needed for doing distillations on most glassware sets. This is very important: a "total immersion" thermometer will give false readings if not *fully* immersed.

In addition to this universal kit, you will probably want to add a larger size boiling flask, say 1000ml or 2000ml. Both are even better. You'll also want a larger separatory funnel. Large separatory funnels are expensive. A solution to this dilemma is to shake small quantities of the mixture in the small funnel and transfer them to a converted jug. (See Figure 3.)

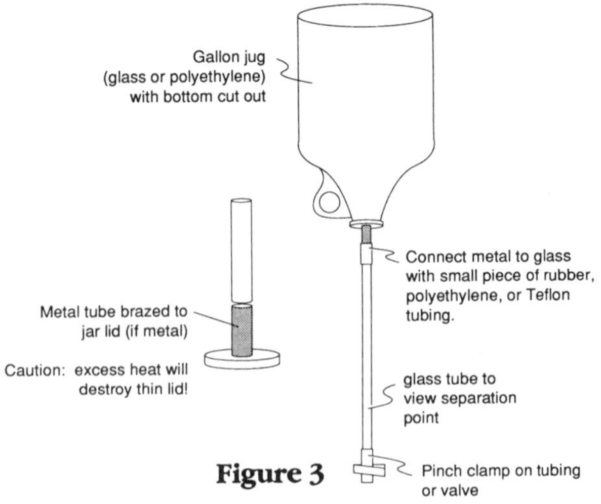

Figure 3

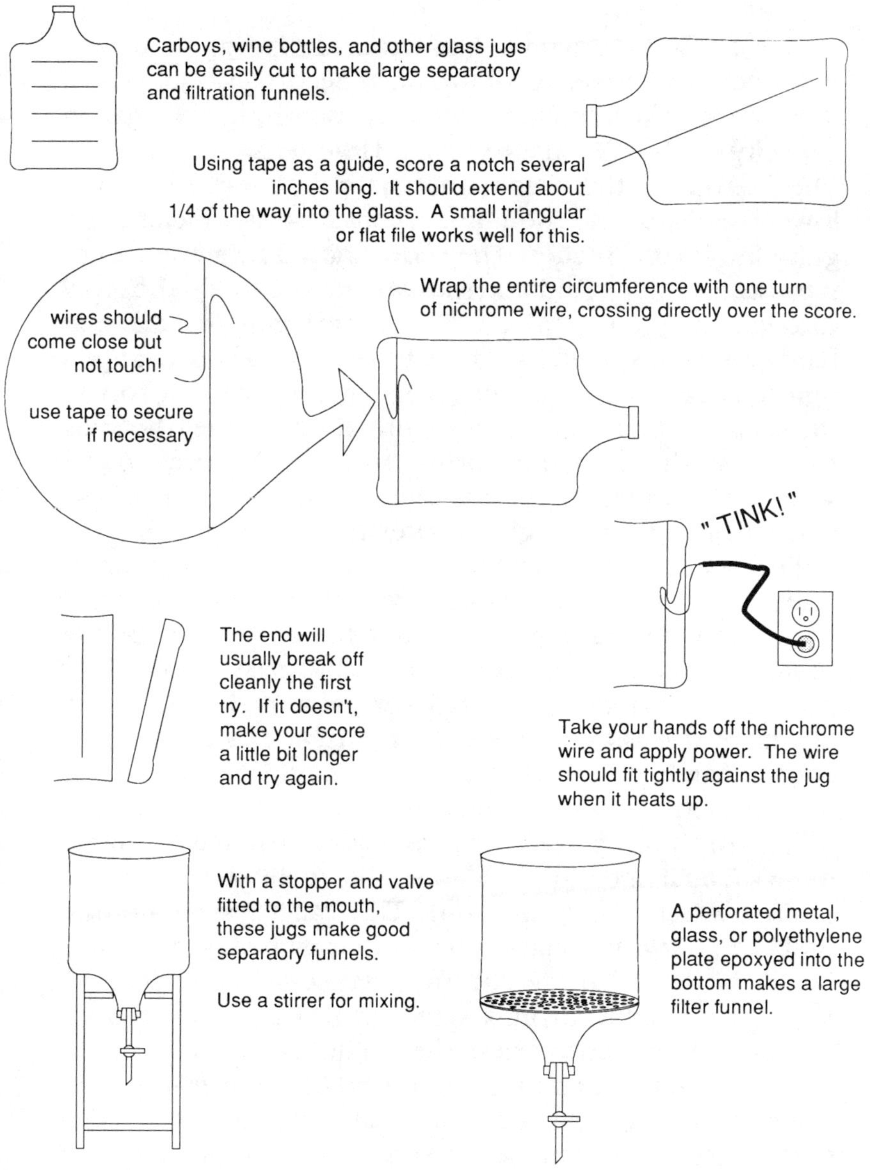
Carboys, wine bottles, and other glass jugs can be easily cut to make large separatory and filtration funnels.
Using tape as a guide, score a notch several inches long. It should extend about 1/4 of the way into the glass. A small triangular or flat file works well for this.
Wrap the entire circumference with one turn of nichrome wire, crossing directly over the score.
wires should come close but not touch!
use tape to secure if necessary
" TINK! "
The end will usually break off cleanly the first try. If it doesn't, make your score a little bit longer and try again.
Take your hands off the nichrome wire and apply power. The wire should fit tightly against the jug when it heats up.
With a stopper and valve fitted to the mouth, these jugs make good separaory funnels.
Use a stirrer for mixing.
A perforated metal, glass, or polyethylene plate epoxyed into the bottom makes a large filter funnel.

Figure 4

For powerful solvents, like tetrahydrofuran, methylene chloride, or acetone, you'll probably need a glass jug. Glass jugs of one gallon capacity, and glass water jugs of 5 gallon capacity (carboys) make excellent large separatory funnels. The bottom of these containers is cleanly cut off as follows: (see Figure 4) the jug is "scored" with a metal triangular file several inches. The score should be straight (use tape as a guide) and extend about $^1/_4$ to $^1/_3$ the way through the glass. A piece of nichrome wire, available at hardware stores, is pulled straight (if coiled) and wrapped tightly once around the jug, passing precisely on top of the score. Overlap the wires slightly (but don't let the ends touch!) so that no gap remains, and apply current to the wire. You can either plug it directly into 110 volt house current or run it through a powerstat. The wire will glow red hot and almost instantaneously you'll hear a soft "tink!" The thermal shock will make a remarkably clean break. If it doesn't work right away, remove the current, make the score longer, and try again after the glass cools. This procedure is remarkably reliable, and is in fact how commercial glass workers cut large tubing as a matter of course. Sanding with silicon-carbide sandpaper will make the sharp edge smooth, if desired.

Turn the jug upside down and you now have a large funnel. You'll need to put an operable drain on the bottom (which was formerly the top). This can be a tight-fitting rubber cork with a glass tube and a pinch clamp, or you could use epoxy putty and fit a stainless steel ball-valve. You'll also need to make a stand for it. Larger size separatory devices are discussed in the scaling up chapter.

For containment and storage purposes, regular glass jars make excellent beakers. Glass salad-dressing and BBQ sauce bottles, as well as jugs can be used in place of Erlenmeyer flasks. The large, 5 gallon glass water carboys are indispensable for storing large quantities of corrosive chemicals. Get into the habit of saving glass jars from the foods you consume.

A wonderful (and expensive) luxury is a "rotary evaporator." These devices take the hassle and wait out of evaporating large quantities of solvents. They spin the boiling flask in a hot water bath under vacuum, making the solvent spread over the entire inside surface of the glass. This increases surface area, and reduces violent, erratic boiling. They have large condensers that quickly recycle solvents into an easily removable receiving flask (to be re-used, of course).

Courses in glassblowing used to be *required* in every chemistry curriculum. Up until 50 years ago, chemists were expected to make all their glassware. Nowadays, this skill is confined to a small handful of specialized, professional glassblowers. Every now and then, a course in glassblowing is offered at some community colleges. If you find one, *sign up for it immediately!* Skills in rudimentary glass working are priceless to the clandestine chemist — especially with the crackdown on sales of laboratory equipment. An excellent book on elementary glassblowing is *Creative Glassblowing: Scientific and Ornamental*, by James E. Hammesfahr and Clair L. Strong. This inexpensive book covers everything from the basics to making exotic scientific apparatuses. The tools required are minimal.

Even if you don't "blow" glass, you can get a few assorted pieces and bend them with a propane torch to make simple stills and condensers. Get soda lime glass to practice with. All laboratory ware used to be made with this glass before the development of "hard" borosilicate glasses. Soda glass can't take extreme thermal shock, but you can work it with an ordinary propane torch. Pyrex is great stuff but you'll need an oxygen-enriched flame to soften it. You can also buy pre-made ground glass joints and stopcocks. These make the fabrication of many items simple. Bethlehem Apparatus Company in Hellertown, PA sells all kinds of glass working tools and kits. Bulk glass tubing, rods, and pre-blown flask blanks can be found inexpensively in the *Thomas Register* under "glass."

Heating, Stirring, and Mixing

This sort of equipment is perhaps the easiest and most economical to construct. Heating mantles are easily constructed using nichrome heating element wire and a suitable cement. Asbestos cement is great. It's also nearly impossible to find since the carcinogenic properties of asbestos have been publicized. Refractory (fireplace) cement or mortar is available from building material and hardware stores. It makes a fairly good substitute. You can also use "kiln" mortar, available from some art supply and ceramics stores. In a larger city, look in the yellow pages under "refractory." Here you'll find many businesses that cater to those who use high temperature equipment and supplies. They have excellent materials for the construction of heating devices, including glass wool, high temperature tapes and adhesives, and a variety of cements. These places also sell fireproof sheets of rigid board (Transite, Marinite) that make excellent liners for fume hoods.

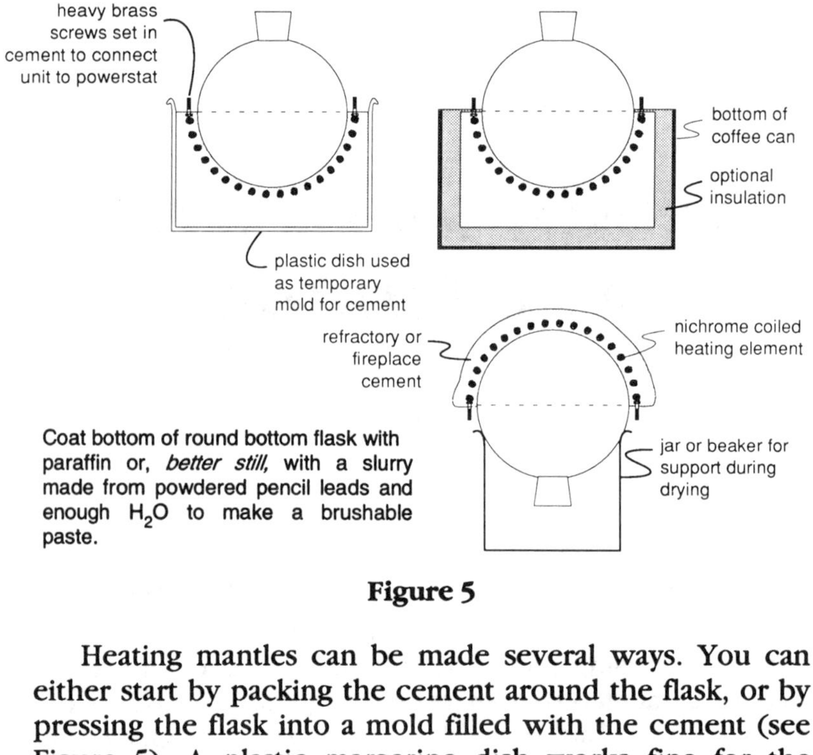

Figure 5

Heating mantles can be made several ways. You can either start by packing the cement around the flask, or by pressing the flask into a mold filled with the cement (see Figure 5). A plastic margarine dish works fine for the latter. The flask can be removed as the cement begins to harden, and the nichrome wire pressed into the surface of the cavity. The flask should then be placed back into the cement as it shrinks during the drying process. Use large brass screws pressed into the cement to connect the nichrome wire to the power cord. The heat can (and should) be controlled by a variable transformer (powerstat). Be certain it is capable of handling the wattage consumed by the length of nichrome wire you have selected. Use a moderately long cord on the heating mantle to place the powerstat away from any flammable fumes. Make sure the connections of the cord to the mantle are tight. A coat of paraffin on the flask will facilitate removal. Better still, is a "mold release compound." There are several types, any of which will work. The *best* for this purpose has graphite in a water based suspension and comes in a spray can. Look for these release compounds at art supply stores and businesses catering to those involved with ceramics and casting.

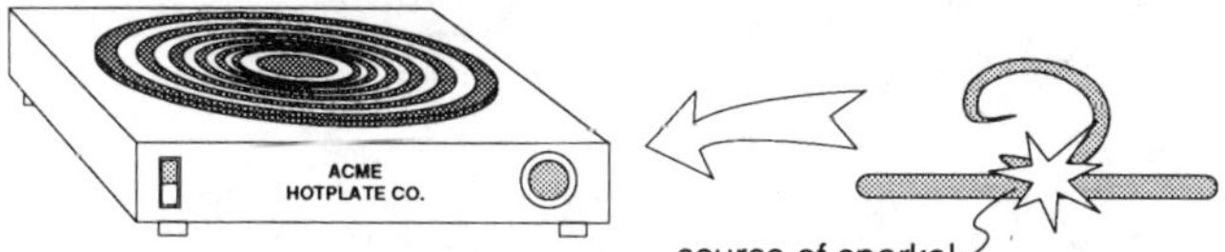

Detail of thermostat: most inexpensive units have a bi-metal, open contact device that shrinks and expands with the temperature. If you're using flammable substances, solder this contact closed (or remove it completely) and control the temperature with a powerstat of suitable size. The powerstat can be located outside your fume hood. Also solder any switches or replace with sparkless mercury types.

Figure 6

Small hot plates can be made sparkless by soldering the internal thermostat closed, and using a powerstat of suitable size to control the heat (See Figure 6). Of course, if you are not working with flammable fumes, there is no reason a regular hot plate won't work.

Don't underestimate a steam bath. They are *excellent* laboratory heating devices. They produce extremely even heat that never exceeds 100 degrees C. This is perfect for drying residual traces of water and solvent out of your product under vacuum. Steam baths also produce no sparks, and are excellent as a heat source for distillation of low-boiling point solvents. Steam baths are easily made using a low profile coffee can (see Figure 7) Cut a hole in the top with tin snips. Make it large enough to allow the desired submersion of the flask or beaker. A steam *generator* can be made by adapting a pressure cooker (see Figure 8) or a heavy metal can (see Figure 9) of most any type.

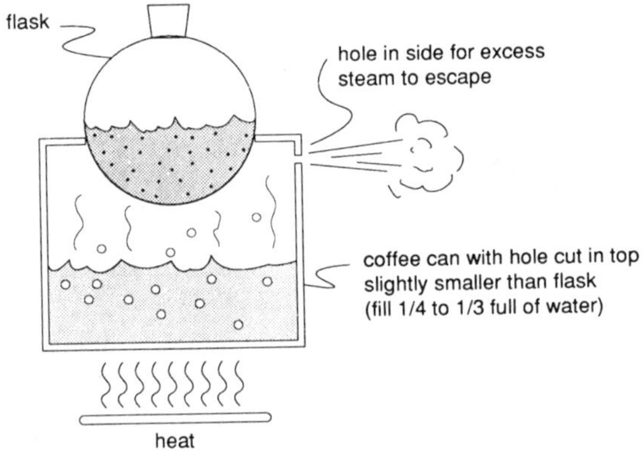

Figure 7

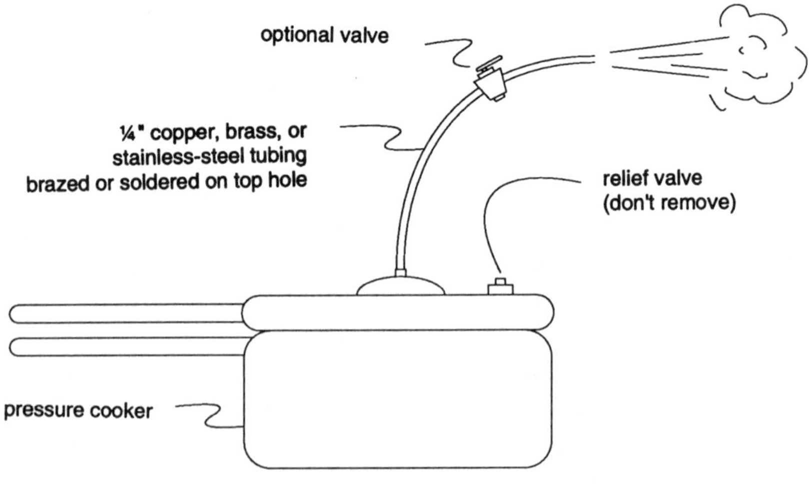

Figure 8

Pipe heating tape can supplement another heating device, and is useful in some circumstances. These are sold in building supply and hardware stores for the purpose of thawing frozen pipes. Most of these tapes have a built-in thermostat that allows operation only below 35 degrees F. Solder the thermostat closed and control the heat with a powerstat. Pipe heating tapes are quite versatile as they can be wrapped around any size or shaped vessel. They do not however, provide the even heat of a good heating mantle. Unless you obtain one made from glass wool or asbestos, they are not suitable for high temperatures.

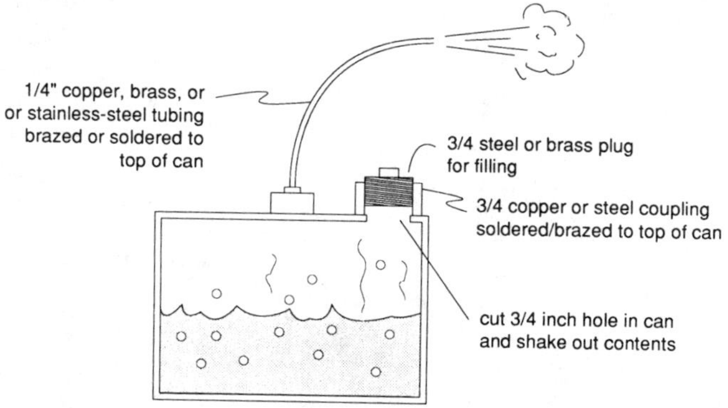

Figure 9

Though a bit messy, oil baths are the method of choice for many heating applications, and they are easily constructed. The high temperature is evenly dispersed over the vessel, eliminating hot spots that cause excessive bumping and foaming. You can instantly control the heat by varying the immersion of the vessel. These baths can be constructed by simply placing an oil container over the heat source (see Figure 10). Another method is to place a nichrome heating element directly into the oil and use a powerstat to control the heat (see Figure 11). A candy thermometer can be clipped to the side to indicate the approximate temperature of the oil. The deep fryers sold in department stores make excellent oil baths. They are compact and transfer nearly all of their heat into the oil. Their internal thermostats make sparks, but you can bypass the thermostat and use a suitable powerstat if you are using it around flammable vapors. For temperatures up to 200 degrees C, mineral, vegetable, or peanut oil are suitable. For higher temperatures, use silicone oil. Silicone brake fluid makes a substitute after some of the lower-boiling adulterants smoke off. Oil baths are well suited to distillation, as they provide a constant, even heat.

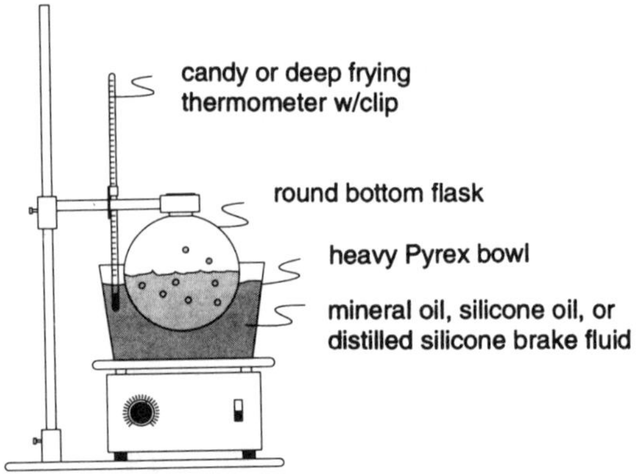

Figure 10

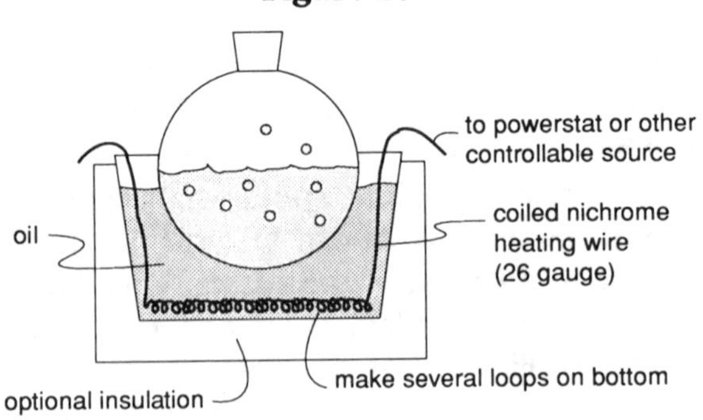

Figure 11

With any oil bath, be certain to support the oil container and other related equipment well. Hot oil all over your legs can ruin your whole day!

Avoid Bunsen burners and other open flame heat sources. They not only supply a source of ignition for fumes, but distribute their heat unevenly. This sharp concentration of heat in one spot can cause glass to break from thermal shock.

Distillations seem to give many readers lots of trouble. Here is my method for hassle-free operations in this endeavor: Keep the quantity small. A 2000ml flask is the largest you should use for most procedures. A 5000 is the absolute maximum, and only for low-boiling liquids. Always use a heating mantle, rather than an open flame. A flame heats one single hot spot on the flask, this makes the boiling quite violent. A heating mantle (either home made or purchased) provides a steady, even heat. You can even blanket the top half of the flask with glass wool for more effective retention of heat. Stir the liquid *during* the distillation. This makes a remarkable difference! The distillation proceeds faster too. The easiest way is with a heating mantle placed on top of a magnetic stirrer. Some commercial heating mantles have a magnetic stirrer built in (expect to pay around 600-800 dollars for one of these gems in the 2000ml size). Another way is to use a 2 neck flask and have a glass or Teflon stirring rod enter through the second opening. You can either stir with your hand (the poor man's method) or you can use a stirring motor. Whichever way you go, you'll be amazed at how much improved your distillations are when done following these guidelines.

Stirring and mixing equipment are easily obtained at secondhand and thrift stores. Garage sales are good too. Old metal blenders cost laboratories hundreds, but they are easy to find second hand for a few dollars. The old milkshake mixers are great for quick immersion into a flask or beaker — a great aid when trying to get some solid powder into solution.

Magnetic stirrers can be easily made from a turntable or tape recorder motor and a coffee can. You can use a ceiling fan speed control on some of these motors, but others require the speed-controlling mechanism in the original device. (See Figure 12.) You might find it convenient to mount the speed controller in the base of the unit. Wadded up chicken wire or a coat-hanger serves to hold the motor in position while the foam sealant dries. Foam sealant adheres vigorously to all surfaces and eliminates the need for complicated shimming and mounting hardware. Epoxy putty, used by plumbers, is an excellent alternative. It hardens to rock hardness in about 5 minutes and can be molded like clay. This great stuff has many uses in the construction of laboratory equipment.

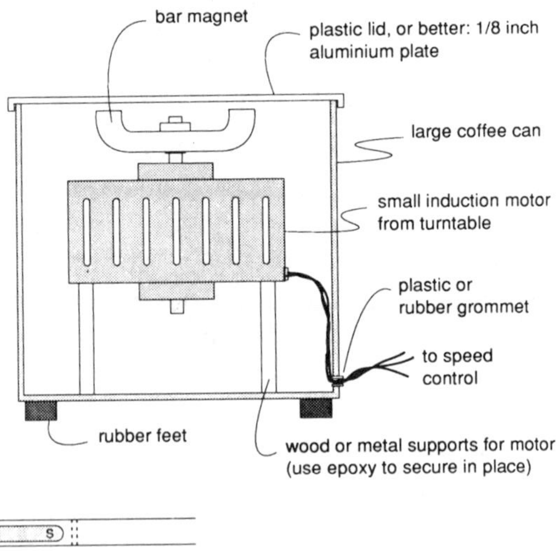

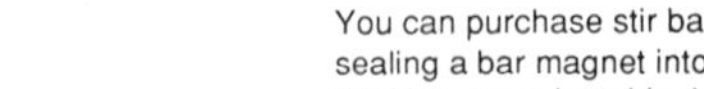

You can purchase stir bars or make your own by sealing a bar magnet into a heavy polyethylene drinking straw (or tubing). Seal the ends with a hot iron or melt them shut with a small flame. You can also use glass tubing, if available.

Figure 12

It's probably best to purchase stir bars. The Teflon coated type is inexpensive and available at scientific supply companies. You can, however, make your own stir bars from sections of polyethylene tubing (the opaque white variety) or thick drinking straws. Melt the ends shut around a small bar magnet. You might even make a "spinning ring" by molding a ridge around the central circumference while the tubing is soft. This feature is found on commercially made stir bars, and is especially useful for stirring large containers with irregular or rough bottoms.

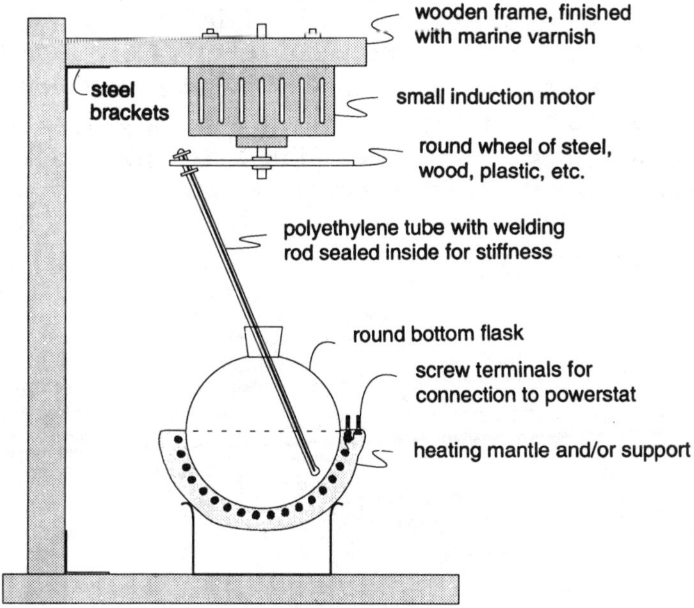

Figure 13

For stirring thick slurries or viscous reactions you will need something more substantial than a magnetic stirrer. A direct drive or "wobble" stirrer serves this purpose. These stirrers are used in the synthesis of the DMT class of drugs, which form a plastic-like intermediate. Don't be misled by the illustration of the wobble stirrer. Your first reaction might be: "Hell, man, I'll just stir it with my hand." But reactions often take hours, and vigorous stirring over the entire period is essential if good yields are to be expected. Construction details of a wobble stirrer are shown in Figure 13. Unless your motor is very small, a reduction is not necessary. Again, a ceiling fan speed control can be used to vary the speed of most small induction motors. If necessary, a small piece of bicycle inner tube can be stretched over the mouth of the flask (the protruding part tucked inward) to protect it from the vigorous movement of the stir shaft. Polyethylene tubes to enclose the stir shaft can be obtained from a "Windex" or other spray bottle. Shown in Figure 14 is a simpler model that can often suffice. It does not vibrate the flask or slosh as violently as the wobble version.

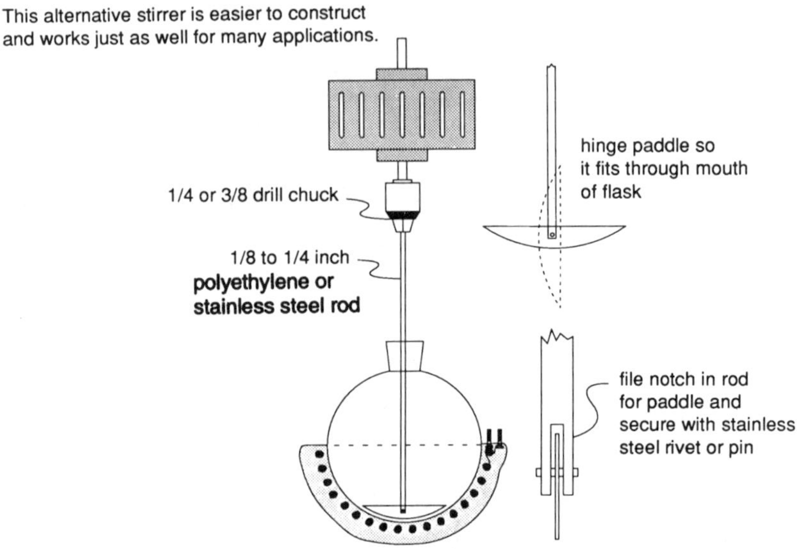

Figure 14

Certain flammable solvents can be used with caution in sparkless mixers such as a blender. Ethanol is okay, especially if diluted with some water. This is done all the time in bars when mixed drinks are made. This procedure is frequently called for when you must grind up a crude plant product prior to extraction. Never do this without good ventilation, and never use ether, acetone, or similar highly volatile solvents. At the very least, use the setup shown in Figure 15. Much better of course is to perform the entire operation inside a fume hood with the blower on.

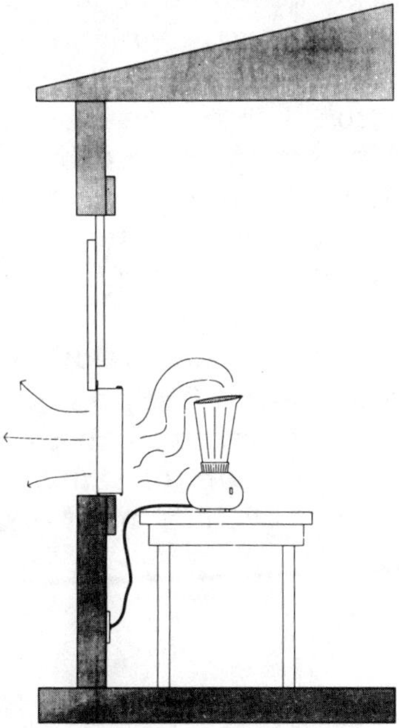

Figure 15

I've mentioned several terms in conjunction with motors in this chapter. I'd like to discuss briefly the various types of motors and clear up some confusion that often arises. AC Motors fall into two broad categories:

universal AC/DC (with brushes) and brushless induction motors. The first type is usually found in small power tools like drills and saws, and has the advantage that its speed can be easily adjusted by use of an inexpensive speed control. Its major disadvantage for the laboratory operator is that the brushes produce sparks that will quickly ignite flammable vapors. Brushless induction motors as a *general* rule produce no sparks. They are divided into several types: "open drip proof," "totally enclosed fan cooled," and "explosion proof." An explosion proof motor produces no sparks; AND it must by definition be able to withstand an internal explosion. Furthermore, it must not allow the internal flame to escape. Be sure you really need one of these expensive motors before you go out and buy one. You can usually eliminate their need by keeping motors out of the area when you use flammable solvents. One place you might consider one is in the exhaust fan of your fume hood, but that will be discussed in detail in the next chapter, on fume hoods.

Induction motors have the disadvantage that it is difficult to control their speed. They rely on the frequency of the incoming line (60 Hz) to establish speed. True, a ceiling fan controller can control *some* small induction motors, but you'll quickly overheat most large ones.

Fume Hoods

Fume hoods are very important to the clandestine laboratory operator. Most importantly, they protect you from toxic material and flammable vapors. However, they also allow the efficient removal of suspicious odors from your vicinity.

Thick sheetrock is an acceptable material for construction of fume hoods, provided it is painted with several coats of epoxy paint or marine varnish. Sheetrock is flame retardant, cheap, and easy to work with. Wood or metal sheetrock studs can be used to reinforce the sheetrock if desired. Use caulk or joint compound to seal the seams up well. Wood can be used as well, provided you line the interior with "stove-board," refractory board, or sheetrock. In fact, any large wooden box can be used provided you protect the interior. Asbestos board is unavailable nowadays, but the ceramic fiber replacements (Transite, Marinite) make excellent building materials for fume hoods. Figure 16 shows the dimensions for a suitable hood from standard 4 x 8 foot stock. You will have to trim the edges to allow for the thickness of whatever material you select. Placement of the baffle is important: one inch off the bottom and two inches from the back. These dimensions produce a hood of the minimum recommended size. A hood about 5 feet wide is the ideal size.

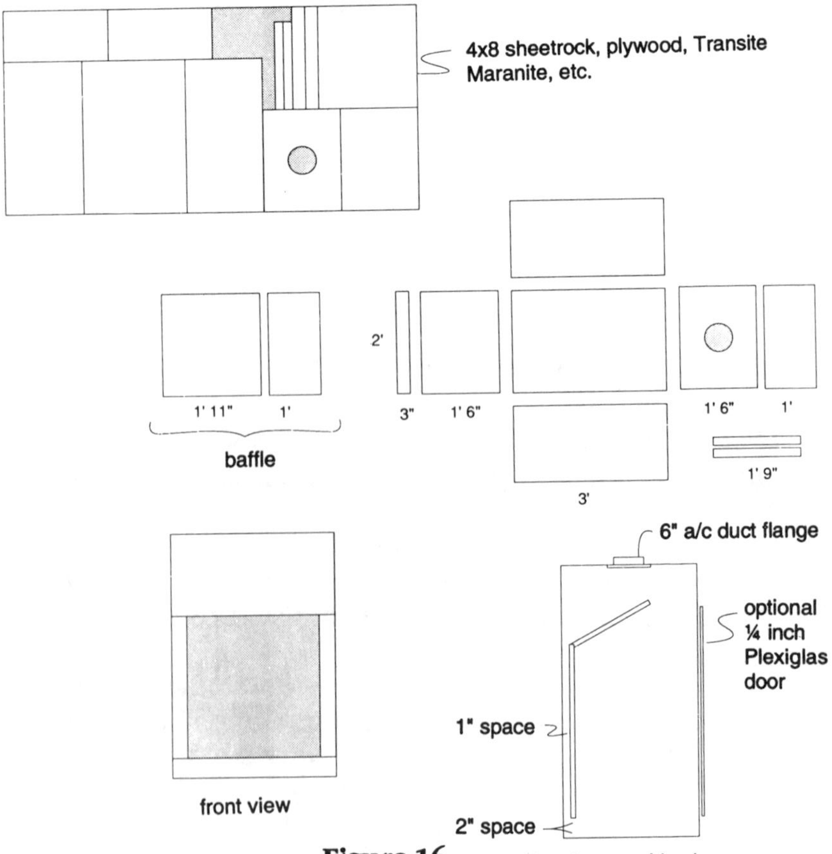

Figure 16

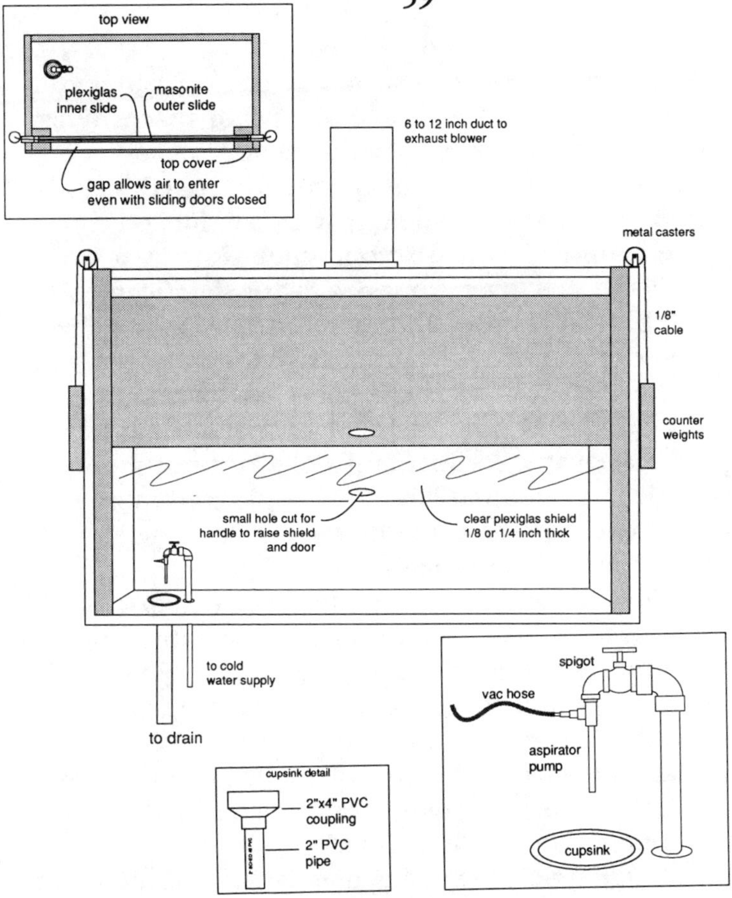

Figure 17

A more elaborate fume hood is shown in Figure 17. This hood has two sliding doors: a clear sheet of 1/4" Plexiglas and an outer solid door that locks closed. I built this hood in a tiny garage and it was a complete joy to work with. The Plexiglas was lowered to within 10 inches or so of the work surface so I could reach in with my hands to work. A light inside provided perfect visibility to an odor free work area, and I was protected from any exploding debris by the Plexiglas. A Halon fire extinguisher was kept mounted nearby and could easily extinguish a major fire in this enclosed, fire-proof space. When not in use, the outer door slid down and locked, completely concealing the contents. It actually looked just like an ordinary workbench when it was all locked up. I strongly recommend you do your chemistry in a hood similar to this. It will lower your risk factor significantly.

A small bar sink is useful mounted inside one of these hoods. You can then have your aspirator pump operating under the hood as well. If you're short on space, a 5 inch piece of 4 inch PVC pipe coupled to a standard 2 inch drain pipe makes an excellent cup sink. You can mount it directly under a spigot and have your aspirator empty into it. Most commercial fume hoods have a "cup sink" very similar to this mounted in them.

A sparkless fan should be used for your exhaust fan. If you really want to do it like commercial labs, use an explosion-proof blower. With one of these, you could safely work a reaction that produced hydrogen or acetylene! 100 cfm is the absolute minimum size. Most large commercial hoods have a blower of about 500 cfm capacity. Figure 18 shows some more details of various blowers and their connection to a fume hood.

Squirrel-cage-type blowers generally make much less noise than their axial (or radial) counterparts of the same size. Furthermore, many squirrel cage blowers have the motor mounted outside the shroud (good ones even have a weatherproof cover for the motor). This makes the risk of ignition (which is fairly low anyway with a brushless, enclosed motor) even less. These blowers are available fairly inexpensively from Grainger, or a similar industrial supply outlet. These blowers are actually quite unobtrusive when viewed from the outside. Drive through a business or light industrial district of your community and you'll see them on just about every building from restaurants to art studios to metal shops.

Best blower for fume hoods

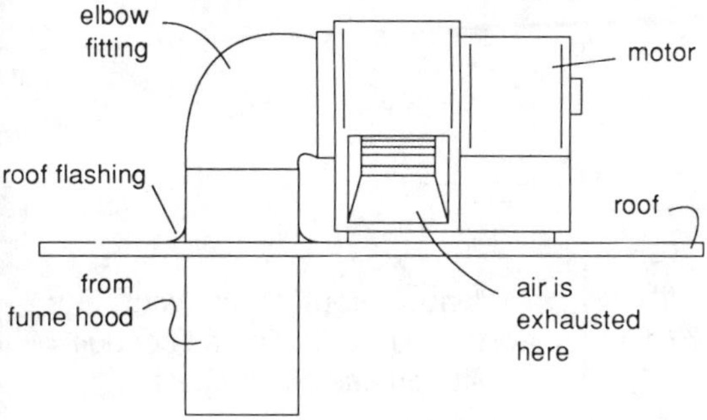

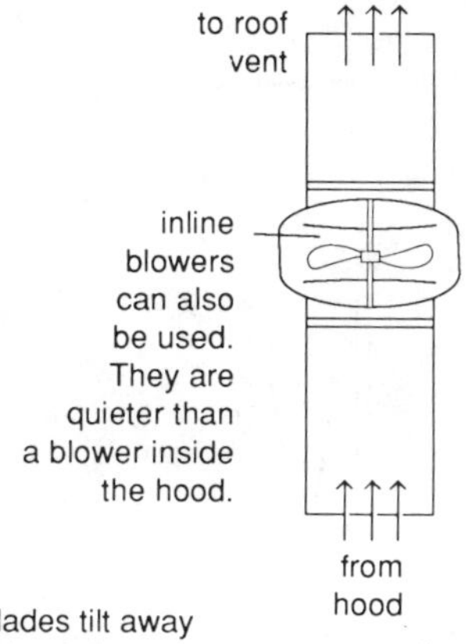

This blower is of the backward incline type. This means the blades tilt away from the direction of travel. This type of blower cannot be overloaded and usually has the motor mounted in a separate, weatherproof compartment. This is the standard configuration for commercial fume hoods.

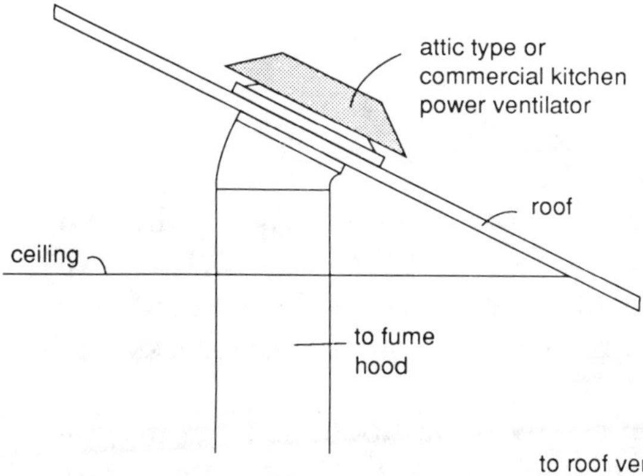

This inexpensive set up works well. It lacks the flow and loading resistance of the backward incline unit, but is fine for many applications. It looks especially unobtrusive. Be sure to use 12 inch duct pipe to prevent excess air resistance that could overload the motor.

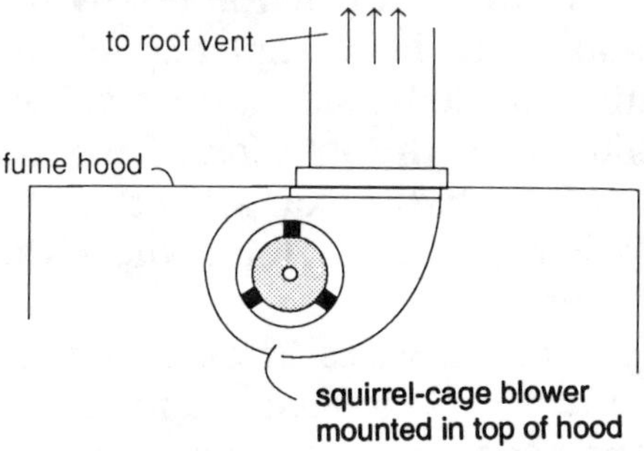

Here is another method. It involves a unit directly inside the hood. The blower must be explosion proof if solvents like ether are used.

Figure 18

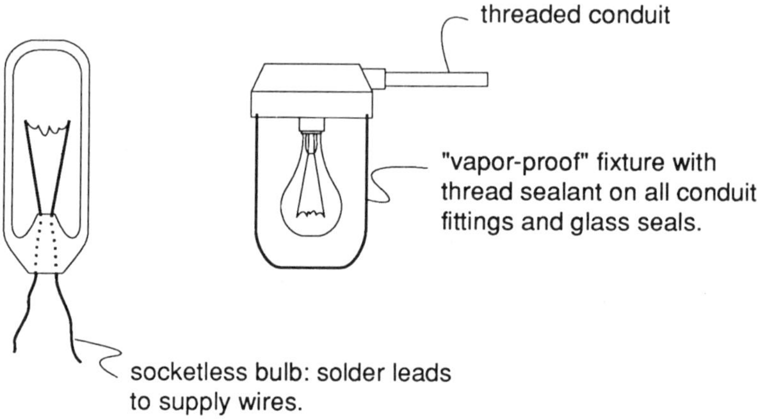

Figure 19

Leave your exhaust fan on continuously so that no smells ever leave your lab. Don't be the idiot that tries to tape all the windows and doors closed — use an exhaust fan and let the fresh air enter through all the cracks and crevices that abound.

In the construction of any fume hood, sources of ignition must be completely eliminated. Make certain any motors used inside are brushless and properly grounded. Illuminate the interior of the hood with a "vapor-proof" outdoor fixture or socketless bulb with soldered leads. (See Figure 19.) Mount the switch on the outside of the fixture.

Run all wires in outdoor-type conduit. The gray PVC variety works nicely and is inexpensive. Eliminate all contact-type connectors such as wirenuts, light-sockets, plugs, etc. Solder all electrical connections and insulate them well. Remember, the slightest spark will ignite many vapors. Keeping the blower on further reduces the risk as the concentration of any flammable fumes is kept quite low.

Exercise *extreme* caution when using ether, even under a hood. The flash point of ether is minus 20 degrees C. This means that even at this temperature, the vapors right above the solvent can be ignited. Keep a fire extinguisher mounted to the wall, within immediate reach.

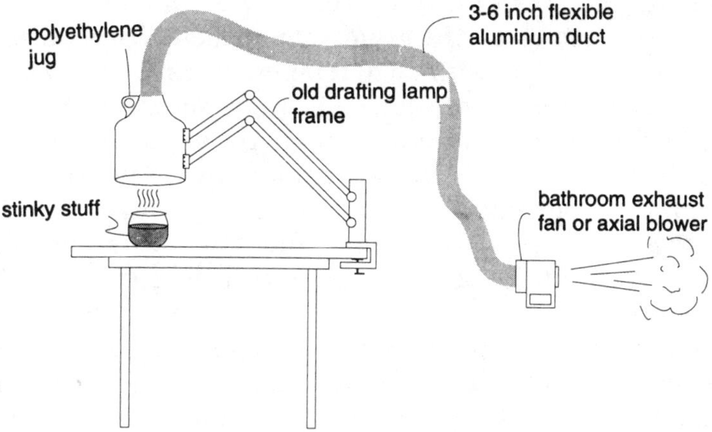

Figure 20

Another useful device is a movable fume hood, suitable for small operations. Construction details of this hood are shown in Figure 20. Use the frame from an old drafting light. Flexible ducting is sold in building supply stores in a variety of diameters. Three inches is the smallest recommended for this hood. Six inches is much better. This device works well for small projects, but it's no substitute for a full-fledged fume hood.

The exhaust of your fume hood blower should be chosen carefully. On a commercial building (with a high roof) or farm, you can simply mount the blower on the roof and let it blow the fumes up into the air. Use the same trick corporate mega-polluters use to obscure their filth: the higher the exhaust, the better. By the time they reach another nose, the odor will be well dispersed and its origin vague. In a house, the vent pipe from the hot water heater or furnace can be used and extended by adding additional sections. If these vents extend high into the air and you are worried about being obtrusive with an extra vent, you can use them as exhaust ducts. Permanently seal all seams in the vent pipe with high-temperature metal tape. (See Figure 21.) A word of caution here: be sure the HW heater or furnace and their pilots are off. To be safe, turn off the main gas cock to these appliances if you're using flammable solvents. This arrangement works well in a basement where the furnace and HW heater are often located. The furnace has a much bigger vent (6-8 inches) as opposed to the HW heaters (3 inches) and should therefore be considered first. I must stress again that using an existing HW heater or furnace duct is an option to consider only if a standard type of blower arrangement is impossible.

Fume hoods are really outstanding. Build one and you'll wonder how you ever did without!

Also excellent for general ventilation are those wind-powered turbine attic vents. Though they lack the airflow needed for most fume-hood applications, they are great for things like your storage cabinets and as a full-time whole-lab ventilator. They consume no energy, are non-sparking, and inexpensive.

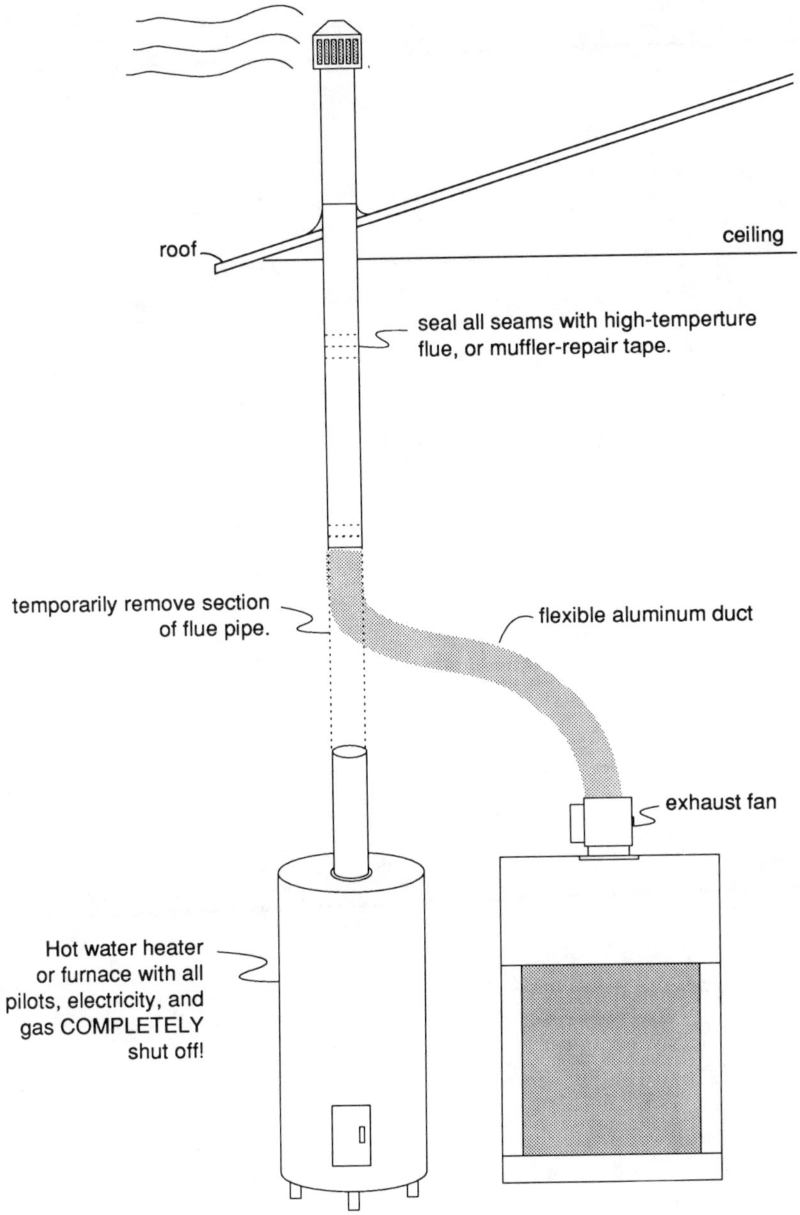
roof
ceiling
seal all seams with high-temperture
flue, or muffler-repair tape.
temporarily remove section
of flue pipe.
flexible aluminum duct
exhaust fan
Hot water heater
or furnace with all
pilots, electricity, and
gas COMPLETELY
shut off!

Figure 21

Miscellaneous Equipment

Most additional equipment can be scrounged from flea markets, auctions, and garage sales. You may have many items already, but haven't associated their use with a laboratory application. Household appliances have the advantages of availability, low-cost, and perhaps most important, unobtrusive appearance.

For non-flammable solvents, an old percolator makes an excellent extraction apparatus for separating crude drugs from plant material, or active ingredients from OTC drugs. Even ethanol can be used if cooling is provided on the lid and good ventilation is available. For moderately flammable solvents, the internal thermostat can be soldered closed and the heat controlled with a powerstat.

Two or three ice bags on the lid provide better condensation of volatile fumes back into the filter (see Figure 22).

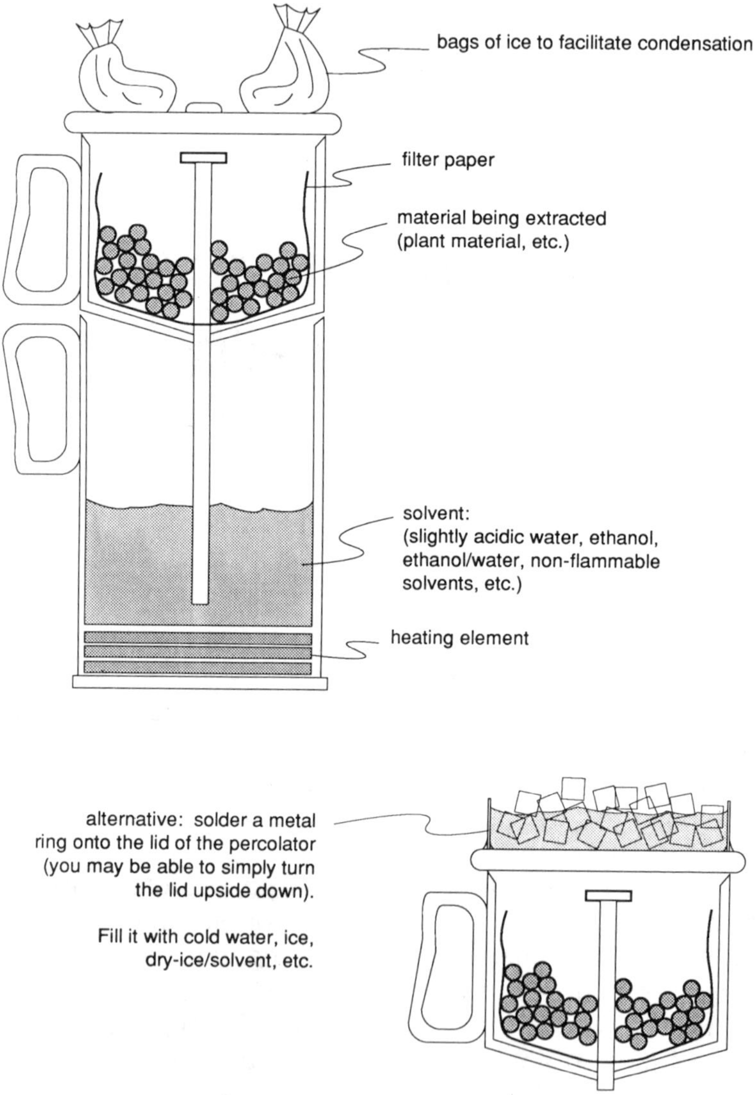

Figure 22

If the percolator is made of brass, copper, or steel, you can solder a small ring of metal to the lid to hold ice or cold water. Epoxy paste will work if the unit is made of aluminum. In some cases the lid can simply be inverted and filled with ice. A dry-ice acetone slush will condense virtually all vapors, but acetone itself is flammable.

The small espresso pots sold in gourmet coffee shops are useful for steam distillation of small quantities (see Figure 23). Steam distillation is useful for the extraction of volatile oils and terpenes from plant material (such as red oil from marijuana leaves and resin).

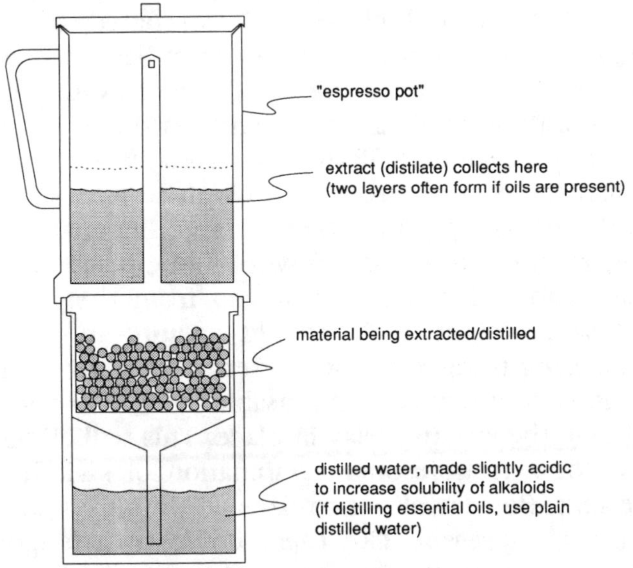

Figure 23

For efficient extraction of many drugs from plant material, fine powdering of the crude substance is necessary. Coffee grinders cost much less than laboratory mills and work nearly as well.

Vacuum pumps are a source of much mail from readers of the first edition. For some reason, people seem determined to make vacuum pumps from refrigerator compressors. In this second edition, I'll share with you my master plans for creating a quality vacuum pump from such a unit, but first I'd like to discuss vacuum pumps in general. I still believe the best vacuum pump for a chemical laboratory is the simple water aspirator. They're cheap, small, sparkless, don't wear out, and flush residual solvents and odors down the drain. With adequate water pressure, they produce a vacuum comparable to many mechanical pumps. Additionally, aspirator pumps have a higher pumping speed (about 7 liters/second compared to 1 liter/minute for a converted compressor). What more could you ask for? This pumping speed is especially important when evaporating or distilling solvents, as the evaporated liquid quickly expands to fill the evacuated glassware.

Mechanical pumps are easily obtained secondhand. Look in the newspaper or browse a large flea market. An old refrigerator compressor can work, but chances are the valves are bad. Why was it removed from the unit for which it was designed? You might acquire an old unit from a *working* refrigerator or freezer. Here is my plan for converting such a device into a usable laboratory vacuum pump: Leave the starting relay in place. This will eliminate the need for a troublesome combination of switches to start the unit. Be careful not to damage the tubes coming out of the compressor. Cut them down to a length of about 2 inches. Turn the unit on and identify the inlet and outlet. Unplug the unit and tip it on its side over a quart sized container so that the outlet faces straight down (see Figure 24). Let *all* the oil drain out (this will take an hour or so), and note carefully how much oil was in the unit. Record this amount, and engrave or scratch it into the case of the compressor (e.g., oil capacity 520 ml). Tip the unit back up and using a funnel replace this exact quantity of oil with "vacuum pump oil." This is available at hardware and industrial supply stores. You will need to change the oil on a regular basis (as with all mechanical pumps) to keep the innards of the compressor healthy. It was designed to run in a closed system.

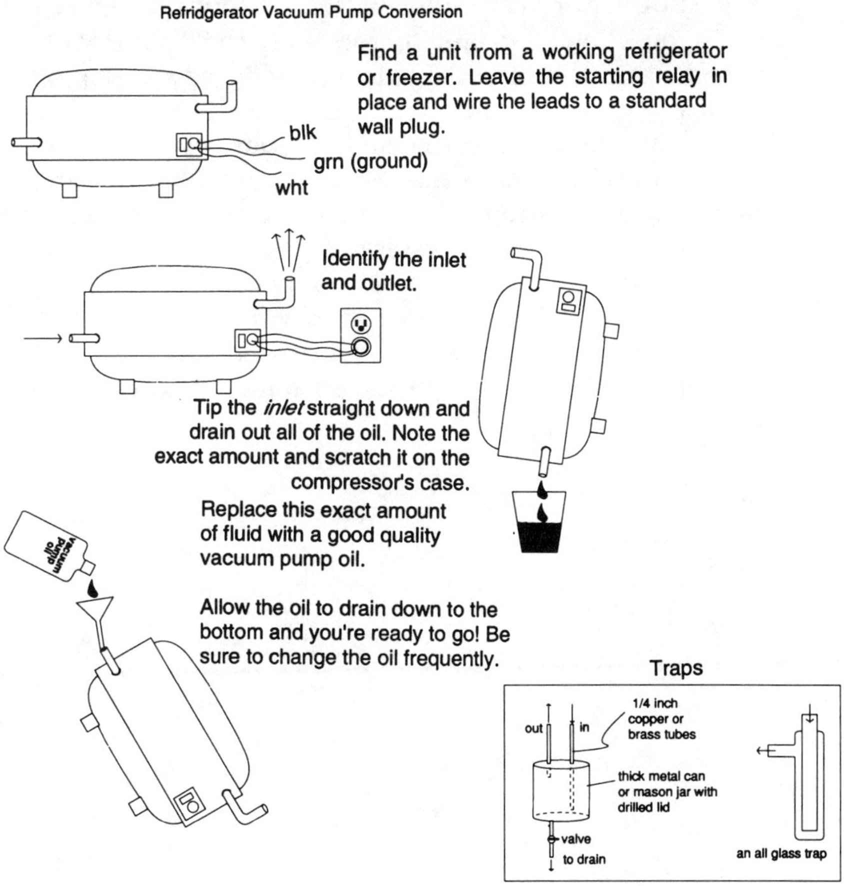

Figure 24

Nevertheless, this pump is excellent for certain purposes, and I wouldn't be without mine for anything. It makes virtually no noise, pulls a high vacuum and consumes no water. It works nicely for vacuum filtrations, drying under vacuum to remove trace amounts of water, and small-scale distillations that don't involve solvents or other highly corrosive vapors. Don't use it at all for evaporating solvents or performing distillations where large quantities of vapor are produced. It will foul up immediately. If you allow the unit to run with the intake wide open to the air, the increased air flow will blow a fine oil mist out the exhaust. This can be avoided by turning the unit on only when it is connected to your system. A few units have an oil separator that automatically filters oil and channels it back to the intake. If you find one of these, all the better, but it's not necessary. A cold trap should be used on all mechanical pumps to condense any moisture and other fumes before they can enter your pump, though you can do without it if you change the oil frequently and avoid high volatiles. Figure 25 shows some additional trap designs.

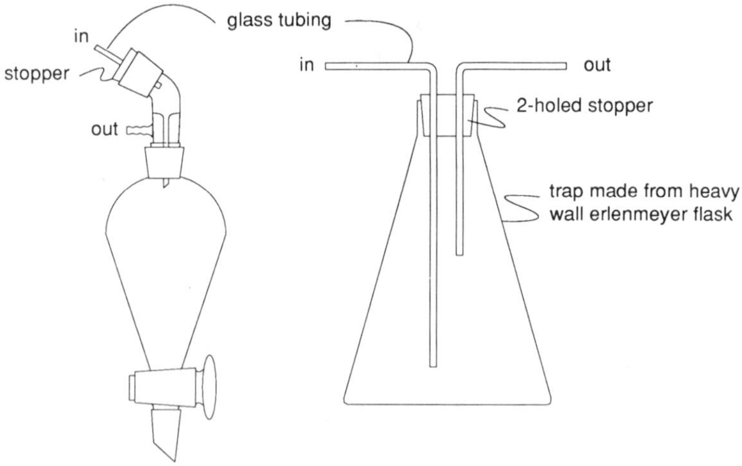

Figure 25

A mechanical pump is a nice accessory, but again, I think an aspirator pump should be the main vacuum source in a clandestine laboratory.

To save water, or if your water pressure is low, you can construct a recirculating pumping station. This station has been completely redesigned since the first edition, and this unit's performance is truly outstanding. Details of this pump are shown in Figure 26.

You'll still need a source of running water to keep the unit cool and flush out condensed solvents as the unit runs. It works quite well, however, and the pump can provide a higher pressure than most any municipal water supply. Use a 5 gallon can, plastic pail, or something similar to house the system. The overflow should have a fitting allowing the attachment of a one-inch or larger drain hose or the unit can be placed in a sink or bathtub. The pump is of the jet pump-type variety, and should be in the range of $^1/_3$ to ½ horsepower. Units made for hot tubs and small swimming pools are also satisfactory; just be sure to check the rated pressure. The pump should provide a pressure of at least 20 psi, but 30 to 40 is much better. Their pressure is usually rated in "feet of head." *Multiply feet of head by 0.4335 to convert to psi.* The use of submersible pumps is not recommended as they raise the temperature of the water, and quickly reduce the vacuum. One pump can usually power two aspirators. The intakes to these aspirators can be connected with a tee for increased pumping speed, or they can be used independently. Increased pumping speed is especially needed when evaporating large quantities of volatile material. As with all aspirator pumps, the colder the water, the higher the vacuum. Adding ice to the reservoir greatly increases the vacuum.

Aspirator Vacuum Station

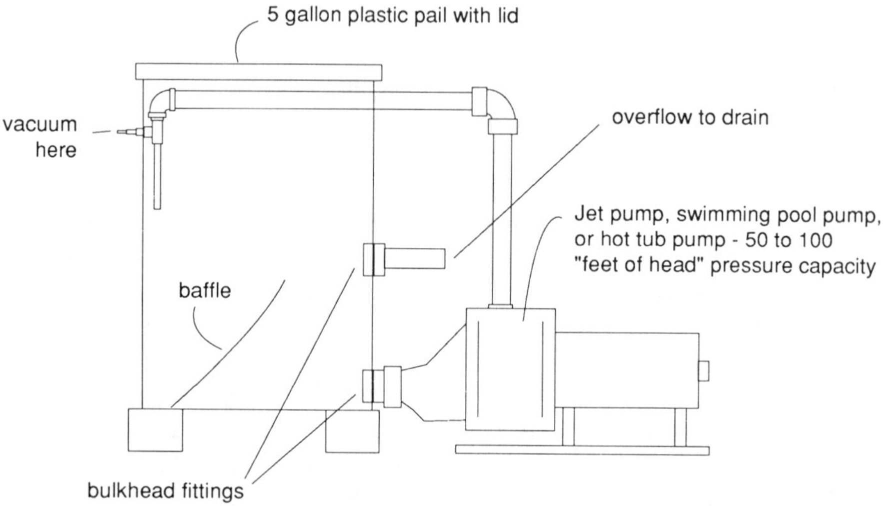

This unit will outperform most any municipal water supply. With 30 psi, it approaches the vacuum of many mechanical pumps. It can handle solvents and other corrosive vapors easily. It can also function out in the country where water pressure is low or otherwise unreliable.

The pail should not seal up air-tight. Leave a small space around the aspirator outlet to allow air to enter. The unit will not drain properly without an air inlet.

The baffle is important. It keeps the bubbly, aerated water from being sucked up by the pump. This would seriously affect performance. An extra lid can be cut into a half circle and wedged into position. Secure it permanantly with silicone.

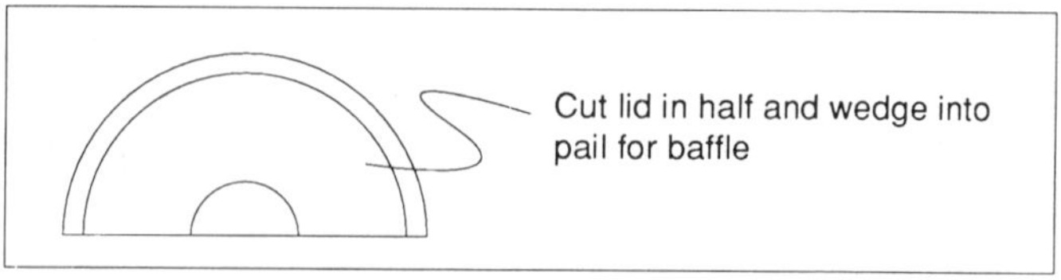

Figure 26

Since the first edition, the price of electronic digital gram scales has come down considerably. I recommend these devices. Accuracy to 0.01g is best. The bare minimum is 0.1g. Old postal scales are useful for rough measurements of large quantities. The old Ohaus "dial-o-grams" are showing up used a lot lately and can be purchased at very reasonable prices. There is no need to feel nervous buying a scale — people from chefs to coin dealers are buying them these days. By all means don't pay the outrageous paraphernalia/head shop mark-ups.

As you scale up to larger and larger quantities, the resolution becomes less important. This is discussed further in "Scaling Up."

Scaling Up

I had originally intended to have a chapter on scaling up in the first edition, but instead decided to emphasize the importance of maintaining a small, unobtrusive operation. Scaling up presents several problems to the clandestine operator. Chemicals bought in bulk quantities immediately flag you as a "manufacturer," rather than an entity performing research. You'll definitely need a larger place — a commercial building with a high ceiling is essential. You'll need more room too — extra space to store your 55 gallon drums of solvents away from your working area. Waste disposal will also be an important dilemma to solve. You can dump some things down the drain, but large quantities of corrosive stuff will quickly trash a plumbing system. Never call one of the chemical disposal services! They will analyze anything you give them (they're usually required to by law), and they have been known to share their information with the police.

Recycling solvents is more important here than ever. A large rotary evaporator with a 5 liter or larger evaporating flask is recommended. It is still important to minimize the amount of precursors you have in your possession at any one time. You'll probably want to keep most of your solvents with you, but never the reagents — keep them in several storage stalls.

You'll probably want to play the part of some industrial-type company to your landlord. A metal plating business, some sort of industrial manufacturer, or other business that would ordinarily have 55 gallon drums lying around.

Odors will be in mega quantity. For this reason your lab should either be in an industrial area that is used to foul-smelling air or out in the country where no one can smell it. A large, roof-mounted exhaust fan is a must. It should stay on all the time — no exceptions.

Fire hazards are particularly amplified when scaling up. Have several large extinguishers in various parts of the building. Fire-proof refractory board should be used wherever needed. Have lots of cat litter handy to quickly soak up any spills before they run out the door or under the wall into the space next door.

Your lab should look the part of some legitimate industrial business on the inside too. It should not be apparent to a stranger that drugs are being manufactured. Put erasable boards up on the wall with bogus project schedules and deadlines. Keep unusual items like glassware out of plain view (under a fume hood with a door is ideal). Don't leave half full jars lying around either. Make it look like legitimate business is conducted there.

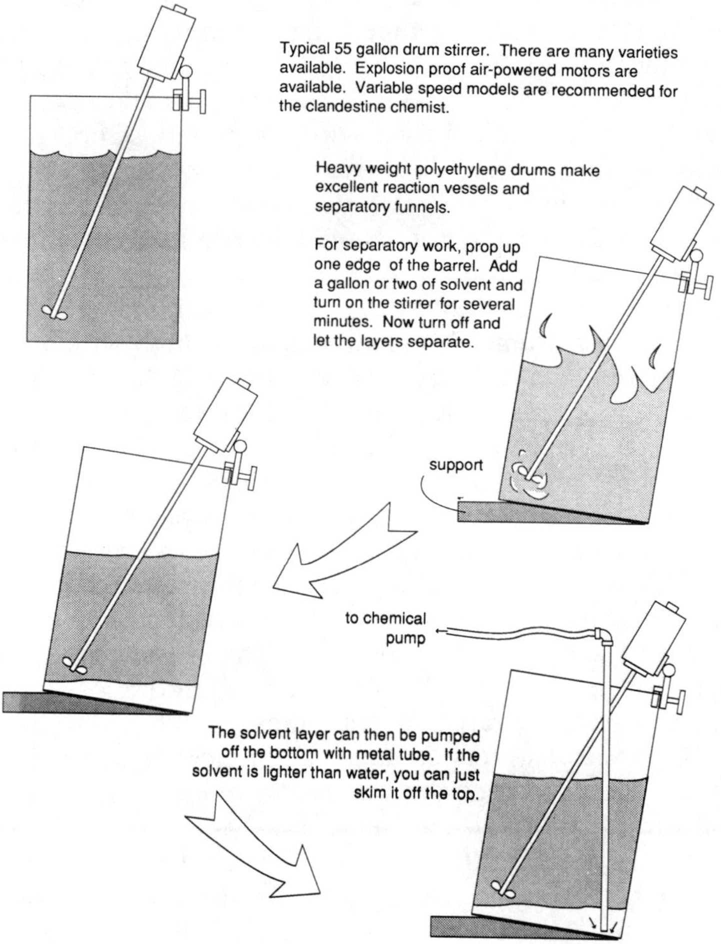

Figure 27

Equipment for large scale production is different. For precise distillations, you can't escape the standard glassware set with ground glass joints, but large sized pieces are available. Look in the yellow pages under "drums" and obtain several heavy-gauge, high density polyethylene containers, 55 gallon size. They are common and available both new and used at low cost. These make excellent reaction vessels when used with a stirrer designed for 55 gallon drums. These big stirrers should be mounted carefully. I once left one unattended and came back the next day to find 50 gallons of would-be product all over the floor! The stirrer was mounted to a sawhorse and vibrated its way across the floor until the stirrer rubbed against the inside of the drum. This made a hole through which I lost what would have been a very rewarding batch. Always mount the stirrer to the drum itself, or anchor it to something that doesn't move. *Heavy-gauge* polyethylene drums further serve to circumvent this problem.

These drums are also used as big separatory funnels. Forget trying to rig up a gigantic funnel with a stopcock on the bottom. Dump your solvent in the drum and turn on the stirrer for several minutes. Turn it off and allow some time for the two layers to separate. The bottom solvent (or water) layer can then be siphoned off into another container. This is repeated several times, just as when using a small hand separatory funnel. Use of clear hose or tubing allows you to detect the separation point. Details of this and stirring are shown in Figure 27.

Instead of a siphon, an air-powered diaphragm pump can be used. See Figure 28 to see what these wonderful pumps look like. They can pump liquids with undissolved solids in them, produce no sparks, and stand up to hard use even when pumping harsh solvents. They are a must for a large operation. You must have a small air-compressor to power it, which can be mounted some distance away. A lawnmower muffler attached to the air outlet on the pump will cut the noise down considerably.

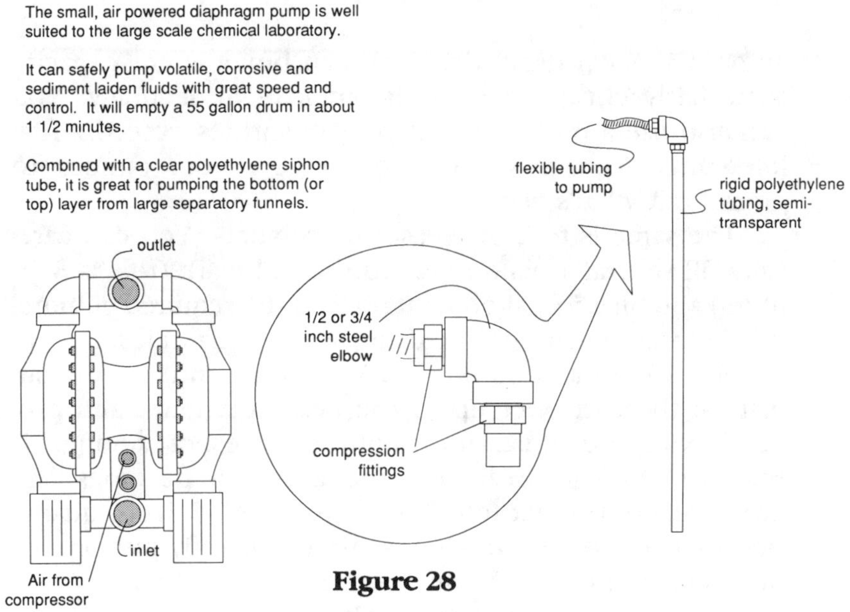

Figure 28

I have not seen any other pump that fits the needs of the chemical manufacturing lab as well as the air-powered diaphragm pump. You'll use it for all sorts of things — emptying drums into the drain, transferring working quantities of solvents from your large drums, etc. They are definitely worth considering! Make sure you get one made of materials compatible with your chemicals. They are available in polypropylene, stainless steel, bronze, and a host of other materials.

As I said before, you'll probably need a large rotary evaporator to process (and reclaim) the large quantities of solvents you use. It is very foolish to use a big fan to evaporate such large quantities into the air. The smell will tip someone off, you'll blow trash into your product, and it's downright wasteful.

Weighing out large quantities requires a slightly different technique. One-hundredth gram accuracy is usually not needed, as total volumes used will be up in the multi-kilogram range. One gram becomes but a minuscule amount in such quantities. You can buy a larger capacity scale fairly cheaply with only single-gram accuracy. You can also use a postal scale if your quantities exceed a few kilograms. You may have to convert from ounces to grams, but what's new?

The same is true of measuring solvents. You can carefully fill several 1 gallon jugs to the full mark (this is 3.79 liters) and fill a 55 gallon container to the required volume. It is helpful to mark on the drum several quantities, say 10, 20, 30, 40, 60 and 80 liters. Then, in the future, you can just fill the container up to the nearest amount and proceed with individual jugs until your exact amount is reached. As with reagents, the accuracy becomes less important as you get into larger quantities. Solvent quantities are even more forgiving, as they're usually just providing a medium in which the reaction takes place. It's always best to start out with the full volumes calculated in scaling up the chemical procedure. It is my experience, however, that you can often reduce the proportionate quantities of solvents used when you scale up. Experiment!

The five gallon glass carboys come to the rescue once again, this time to aid the large scale operator with filtrations. Your final quantities will be in the kilogram range, and it will waste much time to keep emptying a 2000ml vacuum Erlenmeyer flask. Large Buchner funnels are available, and these fit beautifully on top of a carboy with the proper stopper (see Figure 29). You'll need to drill a ½ inch hole in the lower neck area. Glass drill bits are available in hardware stores and look like tiny spades. The trick to drilling glass is keeping it wet to dissipate heat. Use a much lighter pressure than is used for wood bits. I use an ordinary hand sprayer and a cordless drill and usually have a perfect hole in a couple of minutes. It doesn't take a lot of water, just enough to keep the cutting surfaces wet. Rough up the glass around the hole with abrasive paper and attach a brass (or other material) hose bib with epoxy putty. This jug works really well, and seems to be the perfect size for large batches.

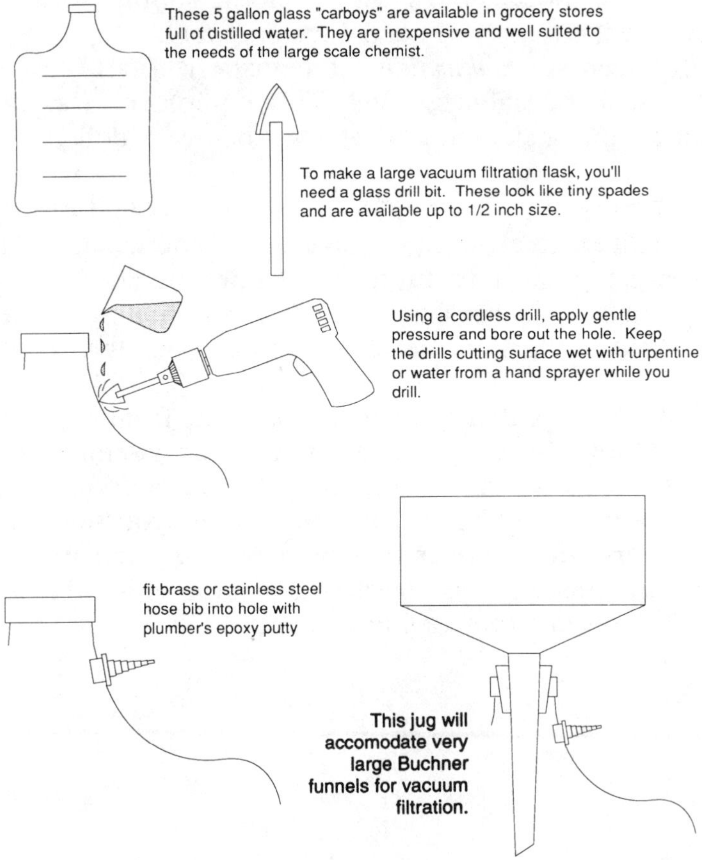

Figure 29

I thought it interesting that several states list "filter funnels" as *watched* laboratory equipment. How ridiculous! Coffee filters work great. If you need vacuum filtrations, you can make your own Buchner funnel out of clay and have it fired. They are also easily fabricated from stainless steel or brass, and brazed together with a torch. Common steel can be used if you have it plated. For the price of a giant Buchner funnel from the supply store, you can buy everything you need, including tools.

I've seen some *excellent* homemade laboratory equipment made of stainless steel. This equipment was built using a MIG welder that cost less than 500 dollars. The owner of this equipment let me try my hand at it. I was very impressed with the ease with which I sealed together two stainless steel tubes — having no experience. A MIG welder can be *very* useful to the clandestine chemist. You can construct unbreakable condensers, boiling vessels, reaction chambers and receiving flasks of nearly unlimited size.

Excellent condensers can also be made from copper or brass tubing of various diameters. You can assemble these with silver solder and a propane torch. It's a good idea to have them nickel plated. This can be done yourself with a car battery, or inexpensively by a plating company. Tell them the condenser is "an aftercooler for an air compressor." They bear a remarkable similarity.

Procurement of Suspicious Items

Next to safety, this topic is perhaps the most important discussed in this book. Chemical companies are now required by law to report the sale of an increasing number of specific chemicals (even some solvents), a list that grows longer each month. I had originally intended to give the reader a list of *all* watched chemicals as of this writing. The DEA, however, is adding chemicals so fast that it would be inaccurate (and create a false sense of security) to present you with "the list." You used to need only look in the *Federal Register* to see what chemicals companies were required to report, but the "emergency scheduling" powers now granted to the Justice Department allow them to add new things without warning. Later in this book, I give you a general list, but beware — it is only a sample! A good journal to read is *Controlled Substances Quarterly*, available at many university libraries. It doesn't list all the items that the *Federal Register* does, but it gives you insight regarding possible future legislation.

We have seen a dramatic increase since the first edition in the difficulty of obtaining required precursors and solvents. This makes the extraction of the necessary chemicals from common sources even more attractive. Neighbors are more aware than ever of telltale signs that drugs are being manufactured nearby. The world's crack-propaganda scene has brought an incredible stigma to the illicit drug world, depicting the illicit chemist as a maniac. This has hurt the clandestine chemist who makes legal drugs and less-harmful illicits. You should browse through the *Federal Register* and *Controlled Substances Quarterly*, before you make a fool of yourself at the local supply store with a paper driver's license.

I was recently in my local scientific store, and a gentleman walked in with ripped jeans and tattoos up each arm:

> "What can I do for you?" said the counter clerk.
> "Eye'd lyke a keeelo of Uhc..ti..Anh..y..dri.." his voice fell apart.
> "A kilogram of what?"
> "Uh... Uhcetic Anhydrite."
> "Acetic Anhydride?"
> "Yeah, that."
> "You'll have to fill out this reporting form, it's required by law. Could I see a photo ID? What did you say your name was?"
> "Uh.... oh, I dun' have my ID, let me seez if it's in thu car..."

Equally inappropriate is to strut in wearing a 3-piece business suit, claiming to be the owner of a large "company" or "corporation." Companies like these don't send someone from their board of directors down to buy chemicals. They have it delivered, mailed, or couriered. If you're needing massive quantities of chemicals, you may feel the need to impersonate a universal, mega-large corporation. In this case, your best bet is probably to make telephone and written contact first, then arrive to pick the stuff up as a courier that works for that big bureaucracy. If you are shopping locally, park across the street for several hours and watch the customers come and go. You'll get a feel for the type of buyer this company is used to dealing with. You might be really surprised!

I hear a lot of talk about "DEA front" companies, set up solely to sell you chemicals then bust you. I personally think their threat is diminishing. I am not saying that they don't exist (I've read about a few court cases), but I personally believe their existence (as of this writing) is slim. There ARE, however, many chemical companies that cooperate fully with the DEA (and other authorities) on a consistent, regular basis.

Establishing a working relationship is more important now than ever. Don't make your first order 200 kilograms of phenylacetic acid. Call them up requesting something specific you *know* they have (i.e., "7mm Teflon tubing" for your "chemical feed pump"). Pick it up, request a catalog, order more and more stuff over time, in larger and larger quantities. Even when you have nursed this relationship to the point of ordering drug precursors, always order other stuff on a routine basis. Credit accounts are often required before you can buy from many vendors. Some may request similar information to set up a "cash account." Someone calling up for the first time to order tubing, or a laboratory labeling kit, or safety goggles IS legitimate; and, the *overwhelming* majority of chemicals sold ARE used for legitimate purposes. You can greatly take the stress and pain out of your first encounter with a new supplier by beginning with something benign. Getting the picture? Just remember, they are required by law to identify the purchasers of many chemicals (and lab equipment in some states), and you should know which ones these are before you are caught with your pants down at the will-call desk. I have included two lists at the end of this book. These are lists of watched chemicals and laboratory equipment I compiled from the lists of several states.

If you've tried to buy chemicals lately, you know that this is becoming one of the most difficult aspects of drug manufacture. Most novice chemists are being weeded out of the business, leaving the more proficient individuals who can synthesize what is needed from more "available" materials. Be sure you insulate yourself well against this weak link in the chain. Always have your chemicals shipped (if purchased by mail) to a place that can sign for the package, and has 24 hour access to you. Then let it sit there awhile. Pick it up early one morning as the sun is coming up. It's easier to blend in and vanish with the morning business crowd at this hour. These mail service centers seem to be getting more popular nowadays. Be sure to check policies concerning customer records and confidentiality. You must also have an answering service that will answer the phone with the name of your company. These service companies are everywhere now and cost little more than a phone line. You can often set up service completely over the phone. That's an additional plus. Get one that can put the party on hold while they try to call you and connect you with the person calling. A digital pager that can display a message from your service can help you return calls quickly, and it insulates you from frequent voice-contact with your service. When you establish an account with your service, consider giving them a false phone number that will never be answered.

Such a phone might be a pay phone in a remote area (or one with no ringer), or the telephone of a business that is never open during daytime business hours. To your answering service, you will only seem like a busy executive who's never home when they call. This will insulate your true identity one step further. To your chemical supplier, you are just hard to catch in your office. Check in with them often and always return calls promptly. Be sure your service is properly instructed: always have them refer to themselves as your "secretary," NEVER as an "answering service."

"Good afternoon. AcmeCo Industries."
"Could I please speak to John Smith?"
"One moment, I'll give you his office..." (No answer.)
"He's out of his office. May I give him a message?"
"Yes, this is David Price with Toxico Chemical. John ordered 2 pounds of Methyl Formamide on Wednesday, and we will not be able to ship it until early next week."
"I see. John will probably want to speak with you about this, I'll have him call you as soon as he returns."
"Thank you."
"You're welcome. Have a nice day."

Don't get stressed out setting up an account with an answering service, bank, or anyone else. Remember, buying chemicals is routine business for thousands of companies from photographers to sheet-metal shops. Call many places, inquire about everything from office furniture to air-conditioning system upgrades — with all these people leaving messages with your service, you're occasional "quotes" from chemical suppliers will blend right in.

Be *immediately* suspicious if you (your answering service) are constantly being called to come pick up a shipment. This is a sure red flag! I had a friend to whom this happened. He had a package shipped to a big freight receiving/forwarding yard in a large city. They kept calling/paging saying "Come on down, we can't hold it forever..." and "...be sure to tell us when you are coming so we can have it ready for you." Sure enough, the package *was* hot. Fortunately, this friend had no criminal record, and no paraphernalia of any type with him at the time, and he was in a city hundreds of miles from where he did his work. They followed him nearly 200 miles to his home town. He was keen enough to notice the surveillance and not make the delivery to his lab or storage space. They finally pulled him over, confiscated the chemicals, and said he had to prove what he was using them for to get them back. It put an end to his clandestine drug business. To this date (years later) he is immediately harassed whenever his name is typed into a government computer, such as at customs, security checks, etc.

Don't freak out when placing orders. Remember, it's not illegal and you're not a criminal for simply ordering a chemical. It's not even illegal to *have* a "chemical laboratory," just to make something in it that *is* illegal. If some company makes it, then someone legitimate is using it. *This is THE secret to obtaining chemicals! Find out who does use it legitimately, educate yourself about that business, and become one of those businesses!* You should often expect a follow-up call asking what you're using chemicals for. Have your stories ready and rehearsed beforehand. Educate yourself on the legitimate use you're claiming for your chemicals. Be prepared to answer *any* question regarding your ostensible business. "What is your market, how long have you been in business, what do you manufacture, what reactions are you working with, etc." Then again, they may not ask you anything at all, and often their "technical service" people are bozos.

It is not suspicious to request rush next-day shipping on chemicals. When I was at a large university, it seemed like every chemical we ordered was a super-rush-we needed-it-yesterday kind of affair. In fact, rush shipping gives them less time to set up some sort of sting, and you know immediately when something is wrong when your package doesn't arrive.

The telephone, in person, or mail? I prefer the mail. If your voice cracks up under stress, definitely use the mail to order what you need. Just be sure you use a good letterhead and envelopes (commercially printed with two or more colors is a must). Your letterhead should have the name of your business, a telephone number, and a fax number (use the number of a fax service company if your answering service does not have one). It should also have an address where you can receive correspondence (NEVER your home or lab), and a *simple* logo that reflects your ostensible type of business. Look at the logos of other big companies if you need ideas. Commercially printed purchase orders are a good plus as well. You can buy these at office supply stores. I always liked the "carbonless triplicate" type with serial numbers. The walk-in chemical supply stores seem to be dropping like flies in the '90s. If you find one you feel good about, then by all means pop in and grab your methylamine and benzaldehyde. Just be sure you're not followed.

Always pay for items with a bank-issued money order or certified check. The convenience-store MOs should be avoided. Of course, you should never use a credit card or personal check. Cash is not easily traceable but looks awfully suspicious.

Always procure chemicals one at a time from different sources, and never while you are manufacturing. Get what you need, store it in a safe place away from your other chemicals, and wait awhile to be sure everything is okay. The best procedure I have used for this type of operation was having several small public-storage stalls rented in different persons' names. These establishments rarely ask for ID, and even then don't scrutinize a fake one closely. Store your chemicals separately in different ones. The "climate-controlled" types are especially well suited. When you need something, you go by that storage space and take exactly the amount you need from your bulk quantity. This way, you are never in possession at one time (other than in your lab, of course) of more than a small quantity of one chemical, and should your operation be busted, you have only a small quantity on hand, with no excess. This is very important in a court of law. The prosecutors love to point out things like, "The defendant had enough precursors to make an additional 2 million dollars worth of methamphetamine. We recommend the maximum sentence of 75 years, your Honor." It has been my observation also that they dump everything that's white powder into a sack and call it "drugs," and dump all liquids into the category of "drugs in various stages of manufacture." So your small-time operation could seem quite massive to a jury that doesn't understand such things.

To a novice chemist, the above procedure may seem extreme. But listen, my friend, the consequences of any misfortune in this era are very, very severe. And setting all this up is easier than you might imagine. You'll only need three or four storage spaces, and you could secure these in one afternoon of work.

Items even hotter than chemicals right now are tablet making machines. Don't be the fool that calls up the manufacturer and tries to order one. They will probably sell it to you, and with it will arrive the biggest barrage of narcs and surveillance you have ever seen. Even manufacturers of dies (which you cannot do without!) are hard to trust now. My advice, unless you really know EXACTLY what you are doing and whom you are dealing with, is to stay far, far away from these menacing machines. Let people further down the hierarchy mess with making tablets. If you insist on making your own, molded tablets are easily made at home and are more than adequate unless you are making tens (or hundreds) of thousands of units.

It can't be done? I didn't write this book to tell you that you can't buy tablet making machines or certain chemicals. Several readers have expressed frustration over obtaining needed precursors, saying it seemed like an impossible task. Well, it can be done, what ever it is, if you want to bad enough. I can't guide every reader step by step through each phase of procurement, as each situation is different. But I'll propose a hypothetical situation, and I'll tell you how I would do it, starting from scratch. Let's say you are convinced that you want to make LSD, a relatively difficult drug to manufacture and procure the necessary items for. Here's what I'd do, knowing nothing:

First, *find out several ways in which it has been successfully made before*. Be sure you know how to spell its full name correctly. Looking in a book about drug abuse, I find that its real name is *lysergic acid diethylamide*. With a computer and subscription to an information service, you could simply do a name-search. If no computer, no problem — just go to the library (a medical or university library is best). *Chemical Abstracts* is a great place to start. It references articles in other publications and provides you with an abstract (short synopsis) of the article, enough to see whether you want to locate the actual article or not. Usually, you'll at least find enough references to other literature. A librarian can tell you other cross-reference periodicals that your particular library may have. *Pharmaceutical Abstracts* is another excellent starting place to locate a broad range of literature. It's also good to simply browse the yearly indexes of various periodicals. Some examples of the hundreds available: *Journal of Pharmaceutical Science, Psychopharmacology, American Journal of*

Pharmacology, Planta Medical — this is just a tiny taste of what's available. This takes time; be patient and don't get discouraged. It takes us all a long time to find out what we want and where to get it.

Anyway, after looking through many articles, I find four different syntheses that I feel I could do. I photocopy them and return them to their place on the shelf. I notice that ergotamine tartarate is the common precursor in three of these, and even the fourth one makes this intermediate after the third step. Great! Time to order? Well, unfortunately, a look through the *Federal Register* indicates that ergotamine tartarate is a controlled substance. In fact, several other ergo-xxx chemicals are also listed. I look back at some of the other syntheses I passed up that did not require this reagent, but conclude after going over them that they're all beyond my capability, require exotic equipment, or produce low yields. Back to ergotamine tartarate! That's what I really need to make, so I look up syntheses for it. Nearly all of them require the use of one of the ergo-xxx chemicals as the starting point, but they are probably all watched to some degree. After more reading, I conclude that the easiest and lowest-risk procedure involves the extraction of ergotamine from dried *ergot*, a dark-purple fungus that grows on rye. Some research on ergot gives me a good idea what it looks like and where to find it. I make numerous field trips to rye fields, finding only minute amounts of the fungus. Finally, I find a commercial source for ergot from overseas (expensive, but better than months trespassing in rye fields), and I stock up, with enough excess to allow for numerous screw-ups while I stumble through the first attempts.

The extraction and conversion (as per the article) of the raw fungus follows — as usual, I get less than expected yields, but I have excess, so there is plenty. As I am squeezing out those last crystals of ergotamine tartarate, I am careful to remove as many impurities as possible, as I still have several steps to go before the final product. When at last finished, I take a break from the long procedure.

The other chemicals seem easy compared to the ergotamine, but I go through the usual precautions obtaining them. I still acquire them from different sources, and order them in conjunction with other benign substances, playing the part of a legitimate industry that would ordinarily buy them in the course of business. The ergotamine is priceless; it stays in an especially secure place. I tear the labels off all of the other jars, referring to them only by the phony names I've written on the lids. This makes them less suspicious should someone stumble onto them, and destroys evidence of where they were purchased. I look for the few solvents needed first at hardware and auto-parts stores. The chemical supply company is always the last resort. With all in hand, and only working quantities in my lab, I am ready to begin a trial run, then proceed with a larger batch.

LSD is more difficult than the norm, so you probably won't have an ordeal this tough to go through. The basic principle is to find a procedure you're comfortable with, then work backwards from the required precursors until you've gotten to a set of chemicals that are not watched closely and that you *can* obtain. Perhaps it is the precursors to the precursors to the precursors. If the drug you're making is obscure, you probably won't have to go much further than making the actual chemicals called for in the procedure. If you're making something like methamphetamine, you'll quickly find that many others before you have thought of the same thing, and you'll have to work way, way back. In the 70s, you could walk right up to the will-call desk and buy phenyl-2-propanone. Today, you can't buy phenyl or acetic *anything*. Even reagent grade acetone is reported! But look around, methamphetamine is more available than ever, so hundreds *are* making it from various things they *are* able to obtain. My hat must go off to the crank chemists — they are a resourceful bunch indeed!

But what if you simply must have a chemical that is reported? Well, don't give up yet. Remember, this list of "reported" chemicals is becoming quite long, and the number of entities buying them is in the thousands per week category. The cost of scrutinizing all these purchases at the federal level and separating them from the legitimate users is very high. You can either set yourself up as a company that has a legitimate use for the reagent, and/or you can fake-ID your way into purchasing what you need. Personally, I don't recommend revealing your true identity to ANYONE in the course of obtaining chemicals.

But *by far* the safest sources of many chemicals are your local hardware, pharmacy and grocery stores. Use laboratory supply companies as a last resort. Many otherwise benign items look suspicious if purchased from a "Laboratory Supplier." These include vacuum drying devices, transformers and thermometers. I stressed this in the first edition, but it holds even more true today. A scant few precursors, and most solvents can be purchased as easily as tomatoes and laundry detergent. Start looking at the ingredients of OTC drugs. You'll find some surprising things! Ephedrine, Phenylpropanalamine, etc. Solvents are the most abundant at hardware stores. Look at the ingredients of the various cleaners and solvents: you'll find acetone, tetrahydrofuran, methyl ethyl ketone, chloroform, methylene chloride, methanol, and nearly everything else. I have used diethyl ether many times, but I have NEVER bought it from a chemical supply house. I have never needed to look further than my corner convenience store, which sells "starting fluid" (my favorite brand was called "Thruster," or something like that). The low boiling point ether is easily distilled in minutes from any other adulterants in the can. Hydrochloric acid is sold for use in swimming pools, magnesium sulfate as Epsom salts, sodium hydroxide in lye, and ethanol in 190 proof vodka. Appendix 5 lists just a few products and the valuable chemicals they contain.

Even more of a gold mine can be found now than when the first edition was written in the form of essential oils distilled from plants. These oils provide the major precursor for a number of the hallucinogenic amphetamines, as well as other drugs. And thanks to a "back to nature" movement, obtaining these oils in quantity is easier than ever. It's interesting that safrole (a precursor of MDA and MDMA) has become a watched chemical since the first edition; and its source, sassafras oil (which is up to 90 percent safrole), is available at my local grocery store for "aromatherapy." Don't overlook plants. Most recreational drugs have a plant-origin precursor somewhere down their line. You'll undoubtedly find references to these during your research of possible syntheses. These sources are often free for the picking.

Drugs have been manufactured for several centuries. But the chemical supply house is a relatively new phenomenon. Chemists used to make *everything* they needed themselves.

The authorities seem hell bent on killing the entire science of experimental chemistry. When I was young, I remember the " Gilbert Chemistry Set" as a very popular Christmas gift. A hundred years ago a "home laboratory" in the basement was common (and encouraged). Now they want your fingerprints if you buy an Erlenmeyer flask. One must wonder what the future holds — will they try to keep people from studying organic chemistry? Censor chemistry literature?

Tablets, Capsules and Other Packaging Methods

After you've synthesized a particular substance, you will need to decide on the dosage and packaging method. You can always stick to plain powder, but it's great to carefully weigh out precise dosages while you are good and sober.

For very small quantities, hard gelatin capsules are often the best choice. They are cheap, and available at drug and health-food stores. They are available in eight standard sizes: 000, 00, 0, 1, 2, 3, 4, and 5, 000 being the largest and 5 the smallest. Capsules are recommended when the amount of substance (drug plus diluents) ranges from 65 to 1000 mg. Lactose is frequently used to increase the bulk of capsulated drugs. A small (5%) quantity of magnesium stearate added to the drug-lactose mixture facilitates easy filling. Prepare a mixture of the drug (corresponding to the number of doses) and lactose necessary to fill the desired number of capsules. Fill only the capsule body, *not* the cap. Using a cotton swab, you can apply a thin film of water to the inside of the cap before placement on the capsule body. Twist the cap as you put it on. This will *seal* the capsule. For larger numbers of capsules, you can make a convenient filler from a block of wood or plastic (see Figure 30).

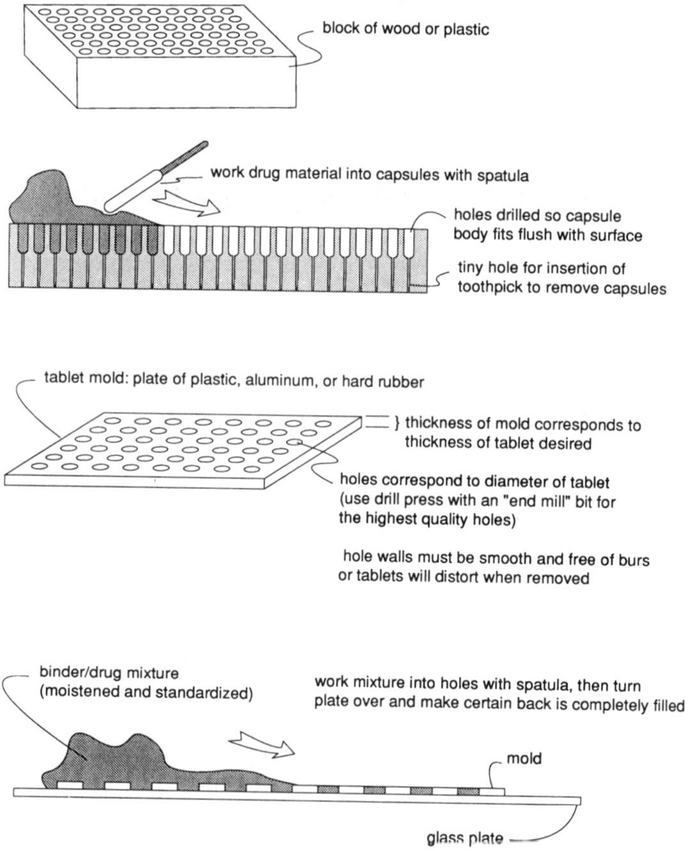

Figure 30

Drill holes such that the tops of the capsule bodies fit flush with the surface of the filler. They should be snug, but not binding. A tiny hole drilled from the other side of each cavity will allow insertion of a toothpick for easy removal of the filled capsules. Use a small spatula or knife to evenly fill (not pack!) the capsules. This well-accepted procedure produces capsules with a remarkable consistency of dosage.

Tablets offer many advantages, especially for the clandestine chemist who sells large quantities. Of course, not all drugs are best put into tablets. But other drugs like the MDA class always seem to find their way into tablet form. With tablets, large quantities of consistent dosages can be produced in a short amount of time. The "operator error" factor is also reduced when stoned people are taking their second helping. Tablets also seem to command higher prices, probably because most persons associate them with "professional" manufacture. Tablets can either be pressed or molded.

Pressed tablets require an elaborate punch and die mechanism. The pressure required varies from 4000 to 40,000 pounds of force. Expensive granulating equipment is needed, and the tablets must have binders and disintegrators added before compression. It takes skill to operate one of these complex machines effectively. I've seen some really sloppy work on the street, with tablets from the same bag varying in thickness 30%. Improperly or inadequately mixed drug and binders also produce grave inconsistencies. However, with very large quantities, there is little alternative. I've already warned you about the risks involved in procuring tablet making machines. There are only a handful of manufacturers, and few qualified buyers exist. I have seen a couple of used units obtained from fly-by-night "brokers." It's just so hard to tell who you can trust. I'm told these two units are both now in DEA seizure custody. Binders for compression machines are best purchased. The best ones are the one-component formulations made with microcrystaline cellulose. They produce a bright white, hard, shiny tablet that breaks cleanly from the dies. Unfortunately, these commercial binders are suspicious to purchase. Caveat emptor.

Molded tablets are considerably easier to work with for the average clandestine operator. These tablets are made by mixing finely powdered lactose with up to 20 percent sucrose (powdered sugar works fine). The more sucrose added, the harder and less brittle the tablet, but more pressure is required. This mixture or "base" is moistened with a 50/50 ethanol (vodka) — water mixture; the ethanol facilitates drying. Moisten the base just enough so that the powder sticks together when pinched between the fingers.

The base and amount of drug corresponding to the number of tablets is worked into a mold. As the tablets just begin to harden, they are gently removed from the mold for final drying. The mold can be made of metal, hard rubber, or plastic. Its thickness should correspond to the tablet's desired thickness. Using a drill press, bore the desired number of holes. An "end mill" will drill a much cleaner hole than a standard drill bit. Sloppy drilling makes the tablets look lopsided, and difficult to remove from the mold. Find a machine shop if needed.

Fifty to one hundred is a good number for a mold. After drilling, grind the chuck-end of the drill (or next larger size if the fit is better) flat. This will be used to gently punch out the individual tablets. If you leave a small, sharp, ridge down the middle of the bit-end, you can make "scored" tablets for easy division into halves (see Figure 31). A light coat of shellac is a nice sealer, and gives a shiny appearance. This sounds odd, but is actually common practice on commercial pharmaceuticals.

Molded tablets don't always have the perfect aesthetics of their pressed counterparts, but they have certain advantages. They are generally more resistant to chipping, and they are easier to maintain consistent dosages in. This is especially true for potent drugs in which the active dose is less than 25 mg.

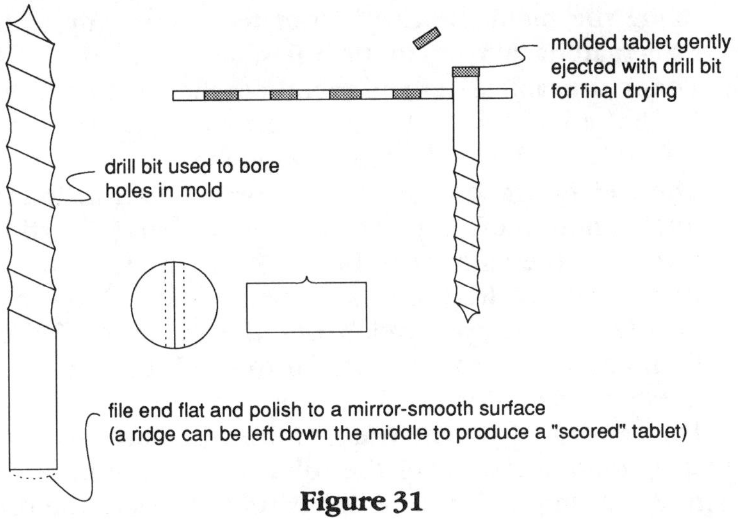

Figure 31

To fill, place the mold on a flat glass plate, and force the moistened base-drug paste into a mold with a small spatula. Now turn the mold over and make certain the bottom is filled also. Allow the tablets to harden a few moments (no longer) and gently eject them with the drill bit end. Let them air dry until hard.

Each drug you package must be standardized to the particular mold you use. Once standardized, you can record the exact formulation to repeat at later times. This standardization is done as follows:

1. Weigh out the amount of drug for the mold. This will be the size of the dose multiplied by the number of holes in the mold.

2. Mix the drug with a quantity of base not quite enough to fill the mold completely.
3. Moisten the base-drug mixture and fill the openings as far as possible.
4. Moisten additional base material (no drug) and finish filling the mold. Be careful not to remove any of the drug material already in the holes.
5. Punch the tablets out and mix them thoroughly.
6. Refill the mold with the mixed base-drug paste. Punch the tablets out and allow to *completely* dry.
7. The weight of these tablets is recorded. Subtracting the total amount of drug substance you initially added gives you the amount of base. This is the standard for this particular drug in this particular mold. From now on, you can simply weigh out the quantity of drug, then add enough base material to reach the weight of the combined, dried tablets.

For *extremely* potent drugs, like LSD, you can apply the drug *dissolved* in a volatile solvent, onto the packaged form. For example, if you dissolve 1000 doses of the drug in 1000 drops of solvent, then each drop contains one dose. You may wish to dissolve each dose in 2, 5, 10 or more drops, depending on the particular potency and solubility of the drug in that solvent. Make certain the solvent does not decompose your drug — this has been common when LSD has been dissolved in aqueous solvents. Also watch for evaporation of the solvent, which will concentrate the drug-solvent solution.

For large packaging of this type, you can use a modified version of the previous method. It requires the use of an accurate balance, however. For example, say you were packaging LSD on blotter cards of 100 doses: weigh a dry blotter card, dip the card with tweezers into the solvent until it is saturated. The hold the blotter card above the solvent and let it drip dry. As soon as the last drop of excess solvent has fallen, weigh the saturated blotter card before the solvent evaporates appreciably. Subtract to find the weight of solvent absorbed by the blotter. You now know that 100 doses are dissolved in this amount of solvent. The cards can now be dipped in the properly prepared solution and hung to dry. This will provide a fairly accurate system for large quantities of potent drugs.

The following formulas and equivalencies may be of use. Be certain to use the same units for all the values when using one of these formulas:

$$\text{number of doses} = \text{total amount}/\text{size of doses}$$

$$\text{child dose} = \text{adult dose} \times \text{age}/(\text{age} + 12)$$

$$\frac{\text{total amount specified in formula}}{\text{total amount desired}} = \frac{\text{quantity of each ingredient in formula}}{\text{quantity of each ingredient in amount desired}}$$

Computers

One tool I have come to rely on since the first edition is a personal computer, coupled with a subscription to several information databases like DIALOG, BRS After Dark, and Knowledge Index (via CompuServe). These searchable databases are goldmines for finding scientific papers describing the perfect synthesis of that reagent you can't seem to procure. They're also *excellent* for finding legitimate uses for the chemicals you must buy, and for finding what common products might contain your needed substances. A quick, 10 minute search can uncover a wealth of information, and you can often print the full text of the article right on your terminal. If not, for a nominal fee (usually 2-7 dollars) you can order copies of the document after you locate it, and they will mail it to you. Often, all you need to see is the abstract, such as when looking for popular commercial uses for a particular chemical. Of course, if you are looking for a synthesis, you're going to want the entire article, along with all pictures, charts, and diagrams.

The learning curve for these services may seem steep at first, but don't get discouraged — they are becoming essential in this day and age. Many of them offer free training seminars that last a full day (usually on a Saturday). Knowledge Index is especially cost effective, and is probably a good one to start with, as their databases include the "International Pharmaceutical Abstracts." DIALOG is the cream of the crop. It's expensive, but nearly every scientific article ever written in recent times is here, often in full text form. A sample search on one of these services might go something like this:

```
1>? begin 121
2> **Now in Pharmaceutical Industry Index**
3>? find (RU-486 and synthesis)
4>      219 RU-486
5>     6278 synthesis
6> S1      4 RU-486 and synthesis
7>? type S1
```

What does all that stuff mean? In the first line, the user tells the service to enter database number 121, the "Pharmaceutical Industry Index." The service confirms, and the user tells them to search in this database for articles that deal with BOTH RU-486 (an "abortion pill") and synthesis. The service responds, saying it finds 219 articles about "RU-486," 6278 about "synthesis," but only 4 that are about both RU-486 and synthesis. The user then tells the service to display these articles. If you want to manufacture RU-486, you'll probably find out how in one of these 4 articles. If not, you'll at least find a great place to start searching for the necessary information, in their bibliographies.

Computers are great for organizing all your notes and records related to your lab. Good records are important to maximizing your yields and procedures. One of the best things about computers is that you can encrypt all of your sensitive information. This is especially important for all of your suppliers' names and addresses. If you are busted, and the police find your records, you can bet they will contact every company you have listed and ask for sales records. All of your notes about procedures, yields, etc. are devastating in the hands of the police. I've spoken briefly with someone who had their computer system confiscated during a bust, and he confirmed that the police meticulously went through his more than 100 diskettes and entire hard drive. If encrypted however, they would have appeared as meaningless garbage to anyone without the proper password.

> *"Sir, you can think what you want, but POOFTER IS the password I used! Your guys must have screwed it up during the raid!"*

I am constantly amazed at how naive people are about their trash. A peek in the garbage is an extremely routine procedure for police. Receipts for solvents and chemicals, broken glassware, chemical-stained gloves, empty bottles (even bottles of "household" chemicals like lye and muriatic acid), shipping cartons with the chemical supplier's address still imprinted on the mailing label, lab notes — leaving any of these in your trash is a potentially lethal mistake that could mark the turning point in your life when you become a convicted felon. Paper shredders are cheap nowadays, and you should use them on EVERYTHING: phone and utility bills, junk mail from lab suppliers, etc. If you live in a metropolitan area, your trash is probably gone through several times each day by transients looking for aluminum cans, etc. These people are usually harmless, but they often pull trash out and leave it all over the sidewalk. Police have definitely been known to pose as transients too, so beware!

The Underground Communications Center

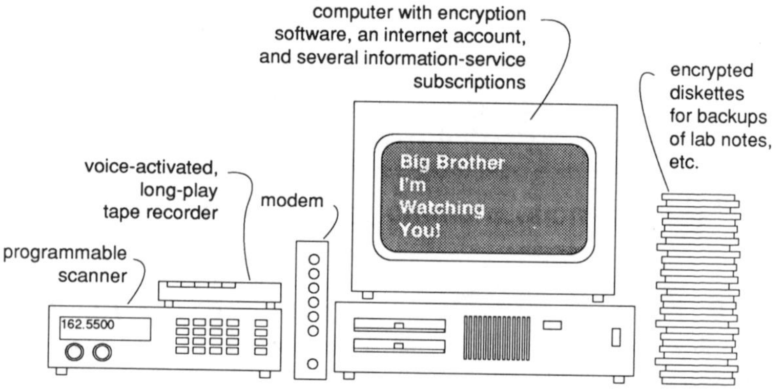

Appendix 1
More Equipment

This easily made pot still works great, quickly condensing large quantites of liquid. Many variations have been made to this classic device. The lid can be rigged with a running water system for cooling. A run off drain can be added to the lid. This will allow the continuous addition of ice without interupting the process to dump the water. A continuous-filling system has also been adopted.

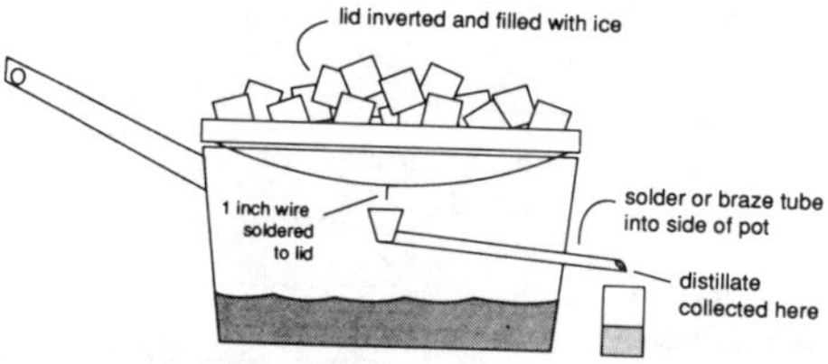

A stainless steel pot is best, but you can also make one from any pan that you can solder. Copper is perhaps the most workable metal, but you should have the completed unit nickel plated for greatest resistance to chemicals.

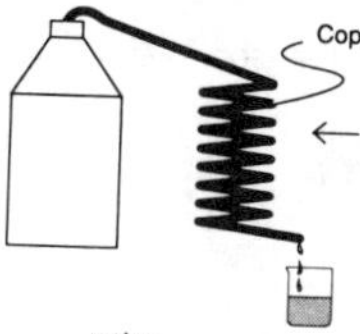

This tin can still was one of the earliest designs. It was used extensively to distill alcohol from fermentation broth for "moonshine." Air provided the cooling. It is a simple, cheap, design on which to come up with your own improvements.

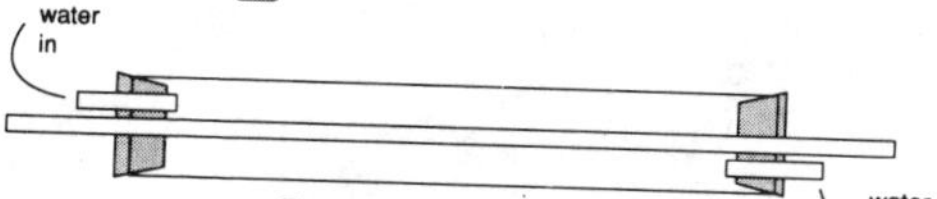

This was once a popular design before the availability of ground joints.

Figure 32

This cabinet works great for drying (or keeping dry) chemicals. The candle provides a slow current of gentle heat through the cabinet and up the flue.

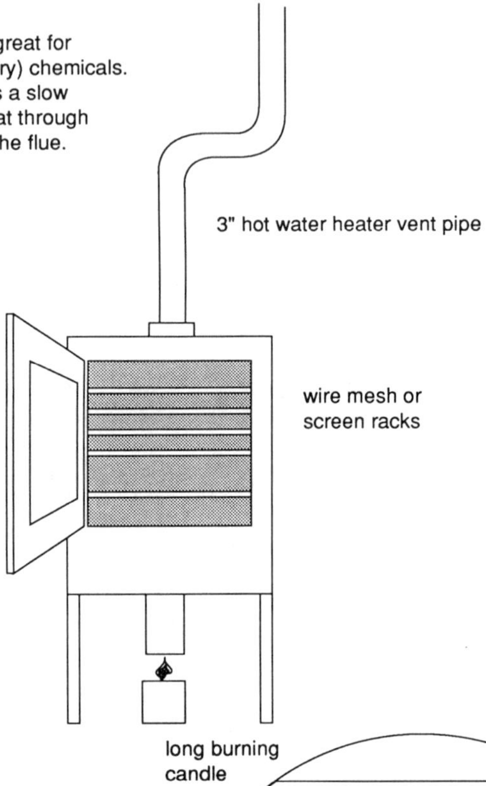

The baffle should be 3 1/2 inches in diameter and 3 inches off the cabinet's bottom. The flame should just reach up into the lower flue.

Cabinet can be constructed of plywood, sheetrock, or sheet metal.

If wood or sheet rock, coat finished cabinet with several coats of marine varnish.

You can also make this cabinet by converting an existing cabinet, or from an old oven.

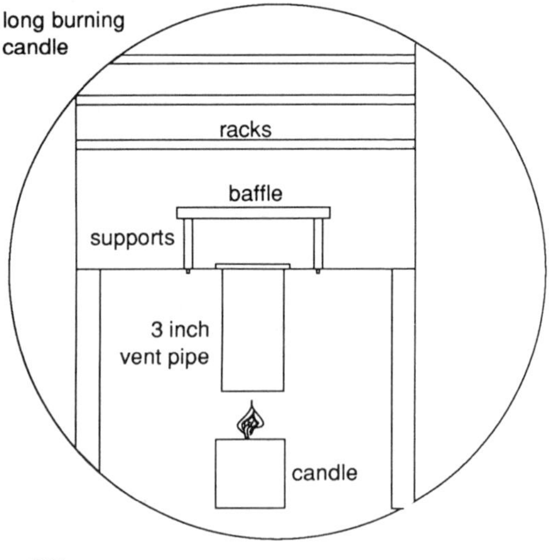

Figure 33

Appendix 2
Watched Chemicals

Ordering any of these chemicals usually says blatantly that you're up to no good:

Acetic Anhydride
Acetone (only reagent grade)
Acetonitrile
Allylbenzene
Amyl, Ethyl, or Butyl Nitrite
Anthranilic Acid
Any Ergo-x compound
Barbituric Acid
Benzaldehyde
Benzyl Cyanide
Bromobenzene

D-Lysergic Acid
Diethyl malonate
Ephedrine
Ephedrine derivatives
Ethyl Malonate
Ethylamine (or its salts)
Formic Acid
Hydroxylamine (or its salts)
Isosafrole
Large quantities of plant oils ordered with other chemicals
Lithium Aluminum Hydride
Magnesium Turnings
Malonic Acid
Methylamine (or its salts)
Methylenedioxy compounds
Morpholine
N-Acetylanthranilic Acid
N-Methylformamide
Nitro compounds
Norpseudoephedrine
Oxal Chloride
Palladium Black
Phenyl-anything
Phenylacetic Acid
Phenylacetonitrile
Phenylpropanolamine
Phosphorous Pentachloride
Piperonyl (heliotropine)
Potassium Cyanide
Pseudoephedrine
Pyridine
Pyrrolidine
Raney Nickel
Safrole
Sodium Cyanide
Sodium Cyanoborohydride

Appendix 3 Watched Laboratory Equipment

Many states now watch the sale of certain kinds of lab equipment. The items below are especially prone to arouse suspicion. I compiled it from the actual lists used by several states:

Buchner Funnels
Capsulating Machines
Condensers
Distilling Equipment
Erlenmeyer, Vacuum Filtration, Round Bottom, Two Neck,
    Three Neck, and Filtering Flasks
Filter Funnels
Heating Mantles
Separatory Funnels

Soxhlet Extraction Devices
Tableting Machines or Presses
Transformers (Powerstats)
Vacuum Drying Equipment

Appendix 4 Legitimate Businesses That Use Laboratory Equipment

Analytical Laboratories
Breweries
Cosmetics Manufacturers
Dairies
Educational establishments (schools, universities, trade schools)
Etching and Plating businesses
Fragrance Manufacturers
Manufacturers of cleaners, detergents, maintenance products, etc.
Medical facilities
Nurseries
Paint Manufacturers

Photo Labs
Research Foundations
Wineries
Foundries

Plus, nearly any industry dealing with cutting-edge technology.

Appendix 5 Common Products And The Valuable Chemicals They Contain

190 proof Vodka	95% Ethanol
Allergy OTC Preparations	Ephedrine
Dexatrim	Phenylpropanolamine
Epsom Salts	Magnesium Sulfate
Lye	Sodium Hydroxide
Muriatic acid	20-30% Hydrochloric Acid
Naphtha	Petroleum Ether
PVC Pipe Cleaner	Tetrahydrofuran
Sinus Decongestant	Pseudoephedrine
Spot remover	Dichloromethane
Starting Fluid	Diethyl Ether

Plants and Plant Products

Calamus Oil	Asarone
Camphor Oil	Elemicin
Hawaiian Baby Woodrose Seeds	Lysergic Acid Amide
Nutmeg Oil	Myristicin
Ocotea Oil	Safrole (90%!)
Sassafras Oil	Safrole

Appendix 6 Recommended Reading

Persons interested in setting up a laboratory will find the following literature interesting:

Psychedelic Chemistry, by Michael Valentine Smith. This book is chocked full of valuable information on all sorts of interesting compounds. Most of the procedures are copied directly from the original scientific literature with additional comments added on synthesis difficulties, dosages, effects, etc.

Psychedelics Encyclopedia, by Peter Stafford. This interesting book isn't really on laboratories or chemistry, but it will introduce you to some of the many plants and herbs that contain hallucinogenic chemicals

Pihkal, by Dr. Alexander Shulgin. This is a gold mine of information on the phenethylamines: synthesis, dosage, effects, etc. The first half of the book is a fascinating glimpse at Shulgin's life.

Creative Glassblowing, by James E. Hammesfahr. This is an excellent introduction into this valuable skill.

Scientific and Industrial Glassblowing. This is a bit more advanced than Creative Glassblowing, dealing only with scientific glassware. It's recently out of print but can be found at many libraries.

The Thomas Register. Nearly any library has this yearly index of manufacturers. Spend an afternoon browsing through it and you'll find sources for just about anything.

The Federal Register. This is the publication the government uses to inform citizens of laws and regulations. You'll find all the nitty gritty details on the controlled substances act and related laws.

Controlled Substances Quarterly. This journal is a good place to see what's going on in the narc world. You'll find valuable clues to upcoming legislation and scheduling of new precursor chemicals.

Grandad's Wonderful Book of Chemistry, by Kurt Saxon. This book is actually the reprints of several vintage books on chemistry, early pharmaceutical preparations, setting up a home laboratory, manufacturing chemicals, and elementary glass blowing. It's a great place to find procedures for making hundreds of chemicals from bare scratch. *Highly recommended!*

The USENET newsgroup "Drugs," for those of you with access to the Internet. This fascinating electronic roundtable is THE MOST progressive and intellectual open discussion on recreational drugs. Hundreds converse daily (many of them Ph.D.'s and specialists in their field) in this dynamic pool.

Catalogs

WW Grainger. This industrial superstore has outlets all over the country (local branches in every major city). They sell pumps, hose, motors, material handling equipment, mixers, exhaust blowers, safety equipment and much more. An excellent technical section is included in the back. They are "industrial," not "scientific" suppliers. They are easy to buy from. 1-800-225-5994 is their national after hours number, but they can tell you the location of your nearest branch.

Fisher Scientific. Ordering from these guys requires a credit account, as they sell chemicals as well. The catalog, however, has nearly anything related to science. It's a good place to look for ideas on building your own equipment. Carpe Diem! 1-800-766-7000. Their address is 711 Forbes Avenue, Pittsburgh, PA 15219-4785.

Cole-Parmer. This company puts out a great full-color catalog with great diagrams, and descriptions of nearly everything they sell. Its another place to look for ideas.

1-800-323-4340. Their address is 7425 North Oak Park Avenue, Chicago, IL 60648.

ACE Glass. This large scientific glassware catalog is a great place to look at what types of things are available. 1-800-223-4524, Vineland, NJ.